T5-CVG-081

Penguin Books

Willing to Listen – Wanting to Die

Helga Kuhse was born in Hamburg, Germany, and came to Australia in 1962. She gained her PhD at Monash University and is now Director of the university's Centre for Human Bioethics. She is the author of many articles and several books on ethics in health care, and co-editor of the international journal *Bioethics*.

Dr Kuhse has been a Consultant to the Human Rights Commission of Australia and to the Victorian Government, and is a member of various professional and hospital ethics committees. She is currently the President of the Voluntary Euthanasia Society of Victoria and of the World Federation of Right to Die Societies.

Married with one adult daughter, Helga Kuhse lives in Upper Beaconsfield, Victoria.

Other books by Helga Kuhse

Should the Baby Live (with Peter Singer)
The Sanctity-of-Life Doctrine in Medicine – A Critique
Embryo Experimentation (with Peter Singer et al.)

Edited by Helga Kuhse

Willing to Listen
Wanting to Die

Penguin Books

Penguin Books Australia Ltd
487 Maroondah Highway, PO Box 257
Ringwood, Victoria 3134, Australia
Penguin Books Ltd
Harmondsworth, Middlesex, England
Viking Penguin, A Division of Penguin Books USA Inc.
375 Hudson Street, New York, New York 10014, USA
Penguin Books Canada Limited
10 Alcorn Avenue, Toronto, Ontario, Canada M4V 3B2
Penguin Books (N.Z.) Ltd
182–190 Wairau Road, Auckland 10. New Zealand

First published by Penguin Books Australia, 1994
10 9 8 7 6 5 4 3 2
This collection copyright © Helga Kuhse, 1994
Copyright in individual articles is retained by the author

All rights reserved. Without limiting the rights under copyright
reserved above, no part of this publication may be reproduced, stored
in or introduced into a retrieval system, or transmitted, in any form
or by any means (electronic, mechanical, photocopying, recording or
otherwise), without the prior written permission of both the copyright
owner and the above publisher of this book.

Typeset in 10/12½ Palermo by Midland Typesetters
Made and printed in Australia by Australian Print Group

National Library of Australia
Cataloguing-in-Publication data:

Willing to listen – wanting to die.

Bibliography.
Includes index.
ISBN 0 14 023775 5.

1. Euthanasia. I. Kuhse, Helga.

179.7

Acknowledgements

I am indebted to many people and several organisations for their help with this collection. Many of the contributors are known to me personally, others I found with the help of some of Australia's voluntary euthanasia societies. For this I am grateful.

My particular thanks are due to those who were willing to write for this collection, even though they knew this would involve the reliving of extremely painful experiences. I thank them for their courage, as I thank those who were willing to defend, on moral grounds, actions that are contrary to existing laws and professional codes of conduct.

I also wish to thank Heather Mahamooth, who transcribed some of the handwritten manuscripts, and Cora Singer, who has helped with proofreading. Finally, I wish to thank Bruce Sims of Penguin Books for the title of the book, and Kathy Hope for making the final production stage such an easy and enjoyable experience.

The editor and the publisher would like to thank the publishers of the following articles for permission to include them in this collection:

'Death by Choice' by Janine Hosking, from *Good Weekend*, 27 May 1988; 'My Mummy's Dying' from *In Search of the Bodgie*, Steve J. Spears, Collins, 1989.

The poem 'On Death', by J. H. Moore, is published by kind permission of the author.

Every effort has been made by the editor, Helga Kuhse, to contact the authors of articles in this collection. She would be pleased to hear from any author she was unable to contact.

Contents

PART THREE *Assuming Responsibility*

Introduction

'Fourteen years ago, I broke the law. Technically, I may have committed murder. Apart from parking offences and civil disobedience ... I am not aware that I have broken the law before or since. In helping my first husband to take his life when it had become intolerable to him, the law says I committed a terrible act. For me, a much more terrible act would have been to watch him deteriorate physically and mentally, to know how unbearable this was for him, and to do nothing.'

Thus writes Mary Mortimer, one of the contributors to this collection. She is not the only writer in this book who admits that she has broken the law to help another person die. There are others as well, some of them writing anonymously, who admit that they have not only been willing to listen to an incurably ill relative, a patient or a friend, who wanted to die, but who were willing to render active assistance. As one of the anonymous contributors writes: 'It's ten years now since I killed my mother. That's right, that's what I did. The hardest thing I've ever done in my life but I had to do it because she asked me to.'

There is hardly a topic that has received greater and more consistent public attention during the last few years than 'the right to die'. Does a person who is incurably ill, who suffers much and wants to die, have the right to bring her life to an end, and is it proper for others to help her in this quest?

For most of the contributors to this collection the answer is 'yes'. They argue passionately and committedly that those who are hopelessly ill not only have a moral right to refuse unwanted medical treatment, or to bring their own lives to an end, but that a compassionate society owes them positive assistance which will allow them to die in a painless and dignified manner, if this is the only way in which they can be helped.

This poses a moral dilemma in its own right: given that direct help in dying is unlawful, how should a husband or wife, a son or daughter, a mother or father, a doctor or nurse, respond to such a request for help? What response is owed to a friend, to a patient, or to a member of our own family who suffers much and who cannot be helped in any other way?

These are the kinds of questions many of the contributors to this collection had to confront in their private or professional lives. Some of the accounts are moving beyond words. They speak of the pain, the anguish, the personal and professional commitment, and love, of one person for another. They also speak of great courage – the courage to challenge existing laws and professional codes of conduct, and the even greater courage to break laws that would have condemned a partner, a relative, a friend, or a patient, to an intolerable life of suffering.

My professional background is in philosophy and ethics, and I have often in the past tried to provide convincing philosophical arguments for the right to die. That there is such a moral right, I have no doubt. While some people would still deny this, I believe the time will come when we will, in great amazement, look back at that period in our history when that right was denied the hopelessly ill – when we failed to respect their autonomy to decide for themselves when it is time to go.

This book is not primarily a philosophical treatise about different moral and religious approaches to suicide or voluntary

2

euthanasia. Much has been written about this elsewhere. If one of the main obstacles to the public recognition of the right to die comes from those who object to suicide and voluntary euthanasia on philosophical or religious grounds, another perhaps even more important obstacle is, I believe, the widespread ignorance about death and dying, and a failure to understand how a civilised society might sensibly and responsibly deal with the requests of the hopelessly ill who want to die. We must add to the abstract philosophical discussions about the right to die the experiences of those who have dealt with dying and death at first hand, and provide a sketch of a professional and social response appropriate for a liberal and pluralist society.

The book is divided into three parts.

Part One focuses on the personal level. In a very moving opening chapter, the journalist Chris Hill explains why he decided to take his life when a hang-gliding accident had rendered him a paraplegic. His account is followed by a plea from his doctor, George Quittner, and his employer, Dick Smith, for social acceptance of, and support for, the right to die.

The next four contributors – all of them women – recount how they have, out of love and respect for the other person, helped to end the life of a member of their family, at that person's request. All have broken the law, three have chosen to write anonymously, but Mary Mortimer wanted her name to appear.

Mollie Collins suffers from multiple sclerosis. She is firmly determined to end her own life, when the disease has progressed to such a state that life has become an intolerable burden. 'Why', she writes, 'are we allowed to put suffering domestic pets to sleep so painlessly and without any trauma, while we ourselves must suffer the indignities of a protracted death?'

The playwright Steve Spears writes angrily about the way

his mother died of cancer, and of the indifference and apathy that followed his requests for political and legal action.

Janine Hosking, a journalist, recounts the tragic story of Cornelis Hus, a quadriplegic, and his friend Wayne McDonald. Following his repeated requests, Wayne shot Cornelis – and then, sadly, took his own life.

Part Two contains accounts by those who care for the ill and dying on a professional level.

Sue Harper has for many years nursed in aged care facilities. Her experience has taught her that proper care for the frail and elderly, and respect for their autonomy, must sometimes include direct help in dying.

Her article is followed by the contributions of three doctors. Roger Hunt, a palliative care specialist, believes that the same principles that underpin good palliative care – namely respect for patient autonomy and the duty to alleviate suffering – must lead doctors to accept active voluntary euthanasia. Paul Komesaroff's article illustrates the complexities of medical decision-making at the end of life; and Rodney Syme recounts how he came to accept the view that doctors have a moral and professional obligation to sometimes give direct assistance to those who want to die.

Until recently, Nicholas Tonti-Filippini was an ethicist at St Vincent's hospital and researcher for the Australian Catholic Bishops. In accordance with traditional Roman Catholic teaching, he denies that we have a right to choose death; he does, however, strongly support the view that people have a right to refuse burdensome life-sustaining treatment. He uses two well-known cases, those of John McEwan and Mrs N., to illustrate the point.

In the final article in this section, Kenneth Ralph, a Minister of the Uniting Church, outlines how he came to accept the view that there are good reasons – respect for autonomy and Christian love – why a committed Christian should support voluntary euthanasia.

INTRODUCTION

In Part Three, the focus switches to the larger question of how a society should deal with the requests of those who wish to die.

Max Charlesworth, a philosopher, argues that in a liberal society personal autonomy, that is, the right to lead one's own life and the corresponding right of others to do the same, is of supreme value. If we take that ideal seriously, then, he argues, we must accept a patient's right to die. To fail to do so is to fail to respect the patient as a person.

In his contribution, Terry Lane supports the liberal ideal, but takes it one step further than others might wish to take it. He argues that *anyone* – not just the terminally or incurably ill – should be able to obtain the means, such as 'a little black pill', that will allow them to commit suicide, if that is what they want.

Pieter Admiraal, a Dutch doctor, is the only non-Australian contributor to this collection. His two cases – those of Carla and Esther – illustrate how doctors can practise voluntary euthanasia openly and responsibly, if they are fortunate enough to be living in a society that permits them to perform this last act of good medical care.

Finally, I sketch the legal situation in the Netherlands and draw some tentative conclusions as to how a country such as Australia might respond to the legitimate pleas of those who are hopelessly ill and want to die.

If there is one idea that permeates virtually every article in this book, it is this one: 'There has to be a more humane way', the title of one of the contributions. It is my hope that the experiences and thoughts recorded in this collection will help us to find this way more quickly. The cost of continued indifference is far too high.

Helga Kuhse
Melbourne, 1994

PART ONE

Wanting to Die

'I wish you could see death as I did, as a release, something to celebrate ...'

Chris Hill

The Note

An open letter to anyone who wants to understand why I've checked out. It's very personal, pretty horrible and perhaps a bit shocking. I hope that those of you who knew me well enough find it unnecessary to read this.

Well, this is it – perhaps the hardest thing you've ever had to read, easily the most difficult thing I've ever attempted to write. To understand my overwhelming sense of loss and why I chose to take my own life, you need to know a bit about my life before and after my accident. Let's take a closer look.

I was born at one of the best times in one of the world's best countries – Australia. I had more than the proverbial happy childhood. Great parents, world travel, a good education and fabulous experiences like Disneyland, swimming with a wild dolphin in the turquoise waters of the Bahamas, riding across the desert sands around the Egyptian pyramids and much more.

Later, after the travel bug had bitten good and hard, I set out on my own adventures. I can remember only a fraction of them, but many rich images come flooding back. I stood on the lip of a live volcano in Vanuatu and stared down into the vision of hell in its throat; I watched the morning sun ignite Himalayan peaks in a blaze of incandescent glory; smoked hashish with a leper in an ancient Hindu temple;

danced naked under the stars with the woman I love on a tropical beach that left a trail of phosphorescent blue footsteps behind us; skied waist-deep powder snow in untracked Coloradon glades; soared thermals to 8000 feet in a hang-glider and have literally flown with the eagles. In Maryland, on midsummer nights redolent with the smell of freshly ploughed earth, I rode past fields lit by the twinkling light of a billion fireflies. I've ridden a motorcycle at 265 km/h on a Japanese racetrack and up to the 5000 metre snowline on an Ecuadorian volcano. And speaking of riding, what haven't I seen from behind the bars of a motorcycle? More than 200 000 kilometres in over a dozen countries embracing everything from some of the world's most spectacular wilderness areas to its greatest cities and vast slums containing millions of impoverished souls.

Along the way I picked up a decent education, including two university degrees, and learnt another language. All this and so much more – more than most people would experience in several lifetimes.

Perhaps most importantly of all, everywhere I've been I enjoyed the support of a caring family, the company of good friends and, more than once, the rewards of being involved in a caring relationship. They – you, if you're reading – are ultimately what made my life as rich as it was, and I thank you.

I was lucky enough to know love, and I indulged in lust. I enjoyed exotic erotica with perhaps more than a hundred women of many different nationalities in places that ranged from the bedroom to a crowded ship's deck on the Aegean Sea, fields, rivers, trees, beaches, cars and motorcycles. There's been ménage à trois's in various combinations and even a few outright orgies. How wonderful to have been sexually active in the pre-AIDS era. I record this not as an exercise in testosterone-fuelled chest beating, but to point out that sex was an important part of my life, and so that you can better understand my sense of loss.

THE NOTE

In short, I once lived life to the max, always grateful that I had the opportunity to do just that, and always mindful to live for today because there may be no tomorrow.

Just as well, it seems. After my hang-gliding accident – how ironic that something I loved so much could destroy me so cruelly – tomorrows were nothing but a grey void of bleak despair. I was paralysed from the chest down, more than three-quarters dead. A talking head mounted on a bloody wheelchair. No more of the simple pleasures I once took for granted. No walking, running, swimming, riding motorcycles, the wonderful feel of grass, sand or mud underfoot, nothing. The simplest of everyday tasks – getting up, having a shower, getting dressed – became an enormous hassle and the source of endless frustration. That in itself was completely shattering physically and emotionally, but I lost so much more than mobility. I lost my dignity and self-respect. I would forever be a burden on those around me and I didn't want that no matter how willingly and unthinkingly family and friends assumed that burden. Every time I had to ask someone to do something for me, every time I was dragged up a damn step, was like thrusting a hot blade into the place where my pride used to be.

All that was bad enough, but there was so much more. No balance. My every action was as graceless as a toy dog nodding in the back of some beat-up car. No ability to regulate my body temperature properly – in a sense I was cold-blooded, more like a lizard than a human being. And without abdominal muscles I couldn't cough, sneeze, shout, blow out a candle or even fart.

Worse still, I couldn't shit or piss. Those body functions had to be performed manually, which meant sticking a 30-centimetre-long silicon tube up my willie four times a day so I could drain myself into a plastic bag, and sticking a finger up my arse every second day to dig out the shit. Sometimes both procedures drew blood. They always made me shudder with revulsion, but I had a powerful incentive to persevere. Autonomic dysreflexia it's called, the potentially fatal rise in blood pressure and excruciating headache that occurs if body waste isn't properly removed and backs up. I had a taste of it in hospital once, and that was enough.

Despite this regimen, there was no guarantee I wouldn't shit or piss my pants in public or wake up wallowing in it. Can you imagine living with that uncertainty? Can you imagine the shame and humiliation when it actually happened? Unbearable abominations that made me feel less than human. For me, it was no way to live.

There's more. I wept every morning when I saw myself in the mirror. I'd become a hunchback with a bloated pot belly above withered legs with muscles as soft and useless as marshmallow. It was an unbearable sight for someone who was once so grateful for being blessed with such an athletic and healthy body. Paraplegia meant that I also had to live with the constant possibility of pressure sores, ugly ulcers that can require months of hospitalisation to cure. They're common. So are urinary tract infections and haemorrhoids. I suffer from both, and they also usually lead back to hospital sooner or later. I would rather die than return to hospital.

Then there was the pain in my shoulder. A damaged nerve meant that two muscles in my left shoulder didn't work and they wasted away, leaving the others to compensate and me with a pain that frequently made simple actions difficult. Then there were swollen ankles, which once meant sleeping with pillows under my feet so they could drain overnight. My chest became hypersensitive, which may sound like fun but meant that I felt like I was wearing an unbearably scratchy woollen jumper over bare skin. And after sitting in the chair for a few hours my bum, which shouldn't have had any sensation, felt like it was on fire. There were also tinea, crutch rot, headaches . . . The list of horrors was endless, and I haven't even mentioned some of the worst ones.

THE NOTE

While at Moorong [Spinal Unit] I began to wake with pins and needles – loss of sensation – in my hands and arms. Sometimes it took hours to pass, and I began to fear losing what little I had left. That was unbearable. Tethering, nerves pinched by the scar tissue formed around the broken bones in my neck, I was told. The doctors talked about tests and surgery on my neck, wrists. Forget it. There was no way I'd return to hospital, let alone for such delicate, radical and debilitating surgery.

All my many pleasures had been stripped from me and replaced by a hellish living nightmare. The mere sight of someone standing up, a child skipping, a bicyclist's flexing leg muscles, were enough to reduce me to tears. Everything I saw and did was a stinging reminder of my condition and I cried constantly, even behind the jokes and smiles. I was so tired of crying. I never imagined that anyone could hurt so bad and cry so much. I guarantee that anybody who thinks it can't have been too bad would change their mind if they lived in my body for a day.

People kill animals to put them out of their misery if they're suffering even a tiny part of what I had to put up with, but I was never given the choice of a dignified death and I was very bitter about that. I could accept that accidents happen and rarely asked 'why me?', but I felt that the legislature's and the medical profession's attitude of life at any cost was an inhumane presumption that amounted to arrogance. And what of the dollar cost? My enforced recovery and rehabilitation cost taxpayers at least $150 000 by my rough count, money that wouldn't have been wasted had anybody bothered to ask me how I felt about the whole thing and what I'd like to do.

I had one good reason for living, of course, and her name is Lee-Ann, the best thing that ever happened to me. Wonderful Lee-Ann, without whom I would have gone insane long before now. But I wept whenever I thought of us together. What future could we have? No matter how hard I worked and how much I achieved, she would inevitably be a nursemaid in a million different ways, and I hated that, no matter that she so willingly and lovingly assumed the burden.

Nor would I condemn her to spend her nights sleeping with a sexless wooden lump twitching with spasm. That's right, sexless – impotent. Stripped of my sexuality, I felt that I'd lost part of my essence, the very core of my masculinity. I was even denied the sensual pleasure of embrace, because from the chest down I couldn't feel warmth, didn't even know if someone was touching me. I love Lee-Ann, but she deserves better than the pointless life I could offer, and I believe that I'm giving her another chance at happiness no matter how much pain I cause in the short term. Someone so desirable – open, honest, natural, loyal, with a great sense of humour and a figure the desire of men and envy of women – has a better chance than most of finding the happiness she deserves, and I hope with all my heart she finds it.

I had other reasons for living, of course – my family and friends. I remember, many years ago, lying on the verandah roof of a colonial mansion in the mountains of northern Burma. A shooting star streaked through the clear night sky and I made a wish. I wished for health, wealth and happiness for all those I loved and cared about. I repeated that wish several times in the following years and was enormously gratified to gradually see it come to pass for most of my family and friends. I'm not suggesting that my wishes had anything to do with their various successes – that was largely the result of their own efforts and the occasional dash of good fortune. But after my accident, even the joy I derived from seeing the happiness of those I cared about went sour for me. Seeing others get on with their lives, doing what I no longer could, was terribly distressing for me. I couldn't live my life vicariously through other people's satisfactions and achievements. I was a self-centred person and I'd always done what I wanted, had my own reasons for living.

Mum and Dad, you often said that you didn't care what I did as long as I was happy. I expect that many of my friends felt the same way. Well, I was terminally, unbearably unhappy with no way out – except death. I know others have come to terms with paraplegia, or even quadriplegia, and managed to lead successful, apparently normal and happy lives. I've met and been encouraged by some of them. I tips me hat to them, for they have done what I cannot. Then again, perhaps I have done what they could not. Four attempts taught me that it takes an enormous amount of courage to commit suicide. Unfortunately, I didn't find the examples of others in my position motivating or inspirational. For me, life as a para was so far from the minimum I considered acceptable that it just didn't matter. It's quality of life, not quantity, that's important.

It's a challenge, many of you said. Bullshit. My life was just a miserable existence, an awful parody of normalcy. What's a challenge without some reward to make it worthwhile?

Despite that, I gave it a go. I worked hard – harder than I ever have at anything – to try and rebuild my life. I tried picking up the threads and doing whatever I was still capable of. I went out to shops, theatres and restaurants, even a concert. I learnt to drive again, and worked. I hated every second of it with a passion I'd never felt before. What good is a picnic when you can't play with the kids and dogs and throw a frisbee? What's the point of going to a gig if you can't dance when the music grips you? I used to be a player, not a spectator, and my new existence (life seems too strong a word) was painful, frustrating and completely unsatisfying.

At least you can still work, some said. Great. I liked my job, the caring, talented and generous people I worked with and especially where we worked. But it was still just a job, and as you all know, I worked to live, not lived to work. Work was never a reason for living for me. And what of the future? Where would I go, what would I do? There's no future for a wheelchair-bound journalist, not one with my interests anyway. I'd never be able to do any of the things, like travel and adventure, that drew me to journalism in the first place and ultimately made the long office hours worthwhile.

I accepted death – embraced it eagerly, in fact, after so many months of the nightmare – without fear or regret. I had a full, rewarding and successful life by any measure, and in my last weeks I couldn't think of a single thing I'd always wanted to do but hadn't yet done. Well, actually, I guess I can think of a few things, but they don't amount to much. I'd always wanted to ride a Harley or drive a convertible Porsche, and I would have loved to have been 'stoked in the green room' – ridden a tube. Surfing would definitely have been the next sport I would have taken up. I've got a pretty good idea of the buzz it offers, and I think I would have liked it. Anyway, death is the last great adventure, and I was ready for it. I wasn't religious – how could anyone believe in a just, compassionate and almighty God after seeing and experiencing what I have? – but I felt quietly confident that whatever lay beyond had to be something more, something better, if anything.

I had one enormous regret, of course. I didn't want to hurt anyone the way I know I have.

I wish it didn't have to be this way. I didn't want to make those I love suffer, and the knowledge that I would bring awful grief to those I least wanted to hurt in the world compounded my own misery unbelievably. I'm so sorry. I hope you can find it in your hearts to forgive me. I wish you could see death as I did, as a release, something to celebrate, and be happy for me. I would rather have thrown a raging party and simply have disappeared at dawn with your blessings and understanding. Of course, it could never have happened that way. At any rate, I thank you all for making my last months as happy as they were, for your optimism and support, for the rays of light with which you pierced my gloom. My condition was permanent; I can only hope your grief fades quickly with the healing passage of time.

Chris Hill
10 February 1993

Statement

I have decided to take my own life for reasons detailed in the accompanying note. It is a fully considered decision made in a normal, rational state of mind and I have not been influenced or assisted by anyone else. Suicide is not a crime and I have the right not to be handled or treated against my will, so I absolutely forbid anyone to resuscitate or interfere with me while I continue to live, unless it is to end my suffering. Anyone who disregards this notice will be committing a civil and criminal offence against me.

In the event that I do not die, I wish to be placed under the care of Dr George Quittner at Mosman Hospital.

Chris Hill

Some Thoughts on the Life and Death of Chris Hill

Chris Hill attended my general practice before he died. I am a family doctor with an average suburban clientele. Chris was anything but average. I enjoy being a doctor. It gives me a special opportunity to nurture and indeed celebrate life.

For me there was something quite chilling about Chris's death – or rather about the response of the detractors, the 'cold blooded' ones, to his death.

Chris's final words soared above his act and made it so much more than just another sad person's suicide. He embodied an ultimate human paradox: those who love life the best are the most capable of ending their own.

Chris's parting letter was filled with the joy of life's experiences from a man who had ventured further than most. It also revealed that his suicide was indeed premeditated in the fullest sense. He had taken special pains over

George Quittner was born in 1952 in Budapest. He arrived in Australia in 1957 as a refugee 'boat person', and experienced a blissful childhood on Sydney's North Shore. In due course he graduated in Medicine from the University of Sydney in 1977, and has been in private General Practice since 1981. He is married and has three children. The founding and only member of 'Medical Dinosaurs', he loves medical practice and hates what the government has done to it.

those who suffer most after a suicide – the people left behind.

I had the privilege to speak with Chris's mother after his death. When I answered her phone call, my hands were sweaty. My immediate response was guilt for not saving her boy. Guilt for allowing his final words to be made public and exposing her great sadness. She thanked me.

The person who loved Chris the most, his mother, had also prayed for his release.

Chris Hill was the best-rehabilitated paraplegic I had ever met. He had an interesting job as a journalist. He drove his own car. He was surrounded by friends and loved ones. He was exceptional in that he even had a devoted woman as his companion.

There was something chilling about the response, of some, to Chris Hill's death.

I did my best to save Chris Hill's life. Despite his objections, I persuaded him to take medication to treat his 'depression'. He gave these mind-altering drugs a fair trial. I admired him for persevering because I knew he hated to take them. Finally he looked me in the eye and said it was pointless. Even with the numbing effect of the drugs, his vitality and his intellect rebelled against his captivity.

I may have been a good doctor but I could do Chris no good.

There was something chilling about his death.

The thing which horrified me about his death was the comment from numerous bystanders: 'How selfish of him', they said. 'There are people worse off than him', they said. Several callers to a talk-back program about him asked: 'How could he do that to his family?' Yet his father, who rang the same program, said he understood.

Chris's death highlighted those cold-blooded people in our community who *wanted him alive*. These are the people who can turn a blind eye to suffering. These are the people who can say 'You can cope with the pain' to a paraplegic.

WILLING TO LISTEN – WANTING TO DIE

I fear most those people who believe they know what is 'good for me'.

Chris died a lonely death. He was without helpers or companions, alone in his car in a remote car park. It was tragic that a man with his disability was denied any assistance with the most important act of his life. His grieving family should have been with him. He should have been in some warm place surrounded by the things which gave him comfort.

Chris died alone, not by choice, but because he was driven there by an inhumane society. The strident voices who 'sanctify life' drove him to an unpleasant death.

Chris Hill – A Salute

Of all of the excellent journalists at *Australian Geographic*, probably the one who most epitomised the aims of the journal and its spirit of adventure was Chris Hill.

Chris spent many years pursuing his twin loves of travel and adventure in Australia and overseas before he joined *Australian Geographic* as a staff writer early in 1988. Long hours in the office did little to diminish his incredible appetite for adventure.

But in February 1992, Chris's life changed irrevocably when a hang-gliding accident left him paralysed from the chest down. He also suffered neck and wrist injuries. In April 1993, having struggled bravely for fourteen months to cope with his situation, he chose to end his life.

He left his family, friends and colleagues a long and moving letter in which he celebrated his

Richard Harold Smith, always known as Dick, was born in Roseville, NSW, in 1944. Businessman, publisher and adventurer, he founded Dick Smith Electronics in 1968 and in 1982 began the quarterly journal *Australian Geographic.*

A keen aviator, Dick has flown many 'firsts' in both helicopter and fixed-wing aircraft, and he and his co-pilot John Wallington recently completed the first non-stop balloon crossing of the Australian continent. In recognition of his sporting, environmental and philanthropic achievements, Dick has won both the Baden Powell Award and the Lindbergh Award.

full and happy life before the accident. He wrote: 'I once lived life to the max, always grateful that I had the opportunity to do just that, and always mindful to live for today because there may be no tomorrow.

'Just as well, it seems. After my hang-gliding accident, tomorrows were nothing but a grey void of bleak despair.'

He staunchly defended his decision to take his own life. 'People kill animals to put them out of their misery if they're suffering even a tiny part of what I had to put up with, but I was never given the choice of a dignified death and I was very bitter about that.'

His death made me think carefully about the controversial subject of euthanasia. It seemed so cruel that the well-meaning restrictions we place on ourselves denied him the right to die as he wanted to, surrounded by the people he loved.

I wonder how many other people with incurable illnesses or soul-destroying injuries are being kept alive against their will – and at what cost to their personal dignity, their families and even the taxpayer.

Chris's letter helped everyone at *AG* to come to terms with his death. We'd watched him working – even from his hospital bed, where he dictated captions for his Lord Howe Island story (*AG* 28) – and, like his family and friends, tried to help him cope.

In the end though, no one could give him back what he'd lost. He wrote: 'I had a full, rewarding and successful life by any measure, and in my last weeks I couldn't think of a single thing I'd always wanted to do but hadn't yet done ... I wish you could see death as I did, as a release, something to celebrate, and be happy for me.'

I salute Chris for his contribution to *Australian Geographic* and for his courage. I hope the time will come when people in his situation will have the right to make their own free decisions about their personal lives with society's blessing.

Anonymous

Anniversary

It's ten years now, ten years since I killed my mother. That's right, that's what I did. The hardest thing I've ever done in my life but I had to do it because she asked me to.

We were sitting at her kitchen table on a Sunday afternoon in July. Mum was just back from a holiday in Hawaii having gone there to get some sun, for a break from the bleakness of Melbourne in winter. 'I don't feel well,' she said. 'It's cancer.'

'Don't be ridiculous, you think everything's cancer because you've had it before and because of Dad.' I was fed up with her always being pessimistic and depressed. My mother looked well, tanned and relaxed from her holiday. She'd brought presents – chocolates, shells and brightly coloured swimsuits for the children. The children had been trying them on and popped

The author emigrated to Australia from Eastern Europe with her family at the age of six. She was educated at state schools and attended university in the sixties. After graduating she has been lucky, to date, to always have paid employment. In the last ten years she has also co-authored a book and edited a national magazine. Her articles and reviews have appeared in newspapers, magazines and professional journals. She is married with children and since the death of her parents has been trying to work out how to fulfil the responsibility of being the oldest generation in her family.

back to parade their new finery for us before running off again to play dress-ups with the clothes in my mother's cupboard.

My mother wasn't a happy woman. She hadn't been happy for the last ten years, not since she was at last able to give up being a machinist in clothing factories, work Mum had always hated. Occasionally I saw flashes of that joyful young mother who used to go dancing every week, and sang about the house, but they were rare, and had become rarer still since my father died. She wasn't unhappy now either, not the miserable depression she'd been in after my father's death.

'I'm going to see Mr Ansell[1] next week. You know, the surgeon who operated on your father. I want a second opinion, from an expert. Those GPs don't know anything. Look how long it took them before they found your father's stomach cancer. Mr Ansell's a lovely man.'

So she was serious about the cancer, there was no other reason for going to Ansell. 'Where's the pain, Mum? What's the problem? You look really well.'

'It's not so much a pain but I'm losing a lot of weight and I've got no appetite and I don't know ... I'm just not feeling right.'

Cancer, cancer, cancer ... maybe it's gallstones or a stomach ache. Surely it can't be cancer in this bloody family again. She's had bladder cancer already, just after I was married and had gone to live overseas. Nobody told me about it until after it was all over. 'We didn't want to worry you ... what could you do from 15 000 kilometres away? It was better you shouldn't know.' I was furious at this betrayal, at their not allowing me to decide for myself whether I was going to worry or come home. What were they protecting me from? How old was she then? Younger than I am now. Forty-four when she had the cancer and she'd been clear ever since, for the last fifteen years.

Of course she thought it was cancer ... who wouldn't in her place? My father had died of it and many of her friends had died or were dying of it so it wasn't surprising that she should be worried. The dreaded crab, the body invaded and made war on by mysterious alien forces, that sense of inescapable fatality, only recently taken over in the most dreaded disease horror stakes by AIDS.

'I don't want to suffer,' she said.

I thought a lot about mortality and how people respond to imminent death in the years after my father died. Over the next three years my only uncle died, one of my two aunts didn't recover from the anaesthetic when she went into hospital for an eye operation, my husband's father died of prostate cancer, my cousin's 2-year-old died of leukaemia, and about half my parents' close-knit group of friends died. We started joking about how all we had to do was point the car in the right direction and it could drive to the Springvale cemetery by itself, like a homing pigeon. My mother carefully read the condolence pages of the *Jewish News* so she would know what funerals to attend the following week. Death was in the air.

'Are they dying because now that they don't need to work hard anymore they don't know what else to do with themselves?' I asked flippantly.

Before my father I'd never seen anyone die or been with someone who was dying. The few deaths of friends were sudden through car accidents, bizarre strokes of fate and bad luck, nothing to do with normality. My grandparents and their whole generation were dead before I was born, exterminated by the Nazis, so there had been no old people for me to watch grow old, sicken and die. In my early thirties with two small children, my focus had been on making and nurturing life. Those years were spent looking forward into the future – being pregnant, giving birth, feeding and looking after growing and healthy children.

Unwell for months by the time his stomach cancer was

finally diagnosed, my father was operated on immediately and had more than half his stomach removed. He improved and my parents went on an overseas trip. Not long after he returned so did the cancer. We were never told by the doctors – maybe they could tell that we didn't want to know – that stomach cancer as far progressed as my father's was a death sentence.

Dad struggled and resisted all the way. He fought death hard with radiotherapy, chemotherapy – the lot. And he would have tried anything else that promised the chance to prolong his life, however briefly. There was talk about some wonder treatment being given by a doctor on a Queensland island but we never spoke about his cancer directly or the fact that we all knew he was dying. My mother insisted on this – he wasn't to know it was cancer, ever. This ridiculous fiction was perpetuated till the last weeks. By then we couldn't break through, though everyone knew that everyone else knew. The family culture implied that if you didn't talk about it, it wouldn't happen; a belief that naming it made it so. Who was protecting who? Who were we shielding from the need to talk about *the end*? None of us would have found it easy but we weren't allowed to even try. How ridiculous this fiction was when at the same time my sister was encouraging my father to make a tape of his life story for his grandchildren. My mother was telling me something about what women think men can and can't cope with, and who really is the weaker sex.

The chemotherapy was terrible – debilitating and dehumanising. 'It knocks me right down,' my father said. I thought it was lucky that he was bald already and had no hair to lose. Every day there seemed to be less and less of him. My mother made him mushes and thin gruels to eat, took him to doctors and treatments, organised a stream of visitors to keep him from thinking, and nearly went round the bend with fear and anxiety. We were all a bit mad during my father's dying, what with the pretence and the fear and not knowing what to do with our anger, our grief and sense of loss and injustice.

My sister got married earlier than she'd planned, so that my father could be there. My father, a skeleton at the wedding, died three months later. 'Don't let them take me to hospital,' he begged, so my mother looked after him at home. She bathed him, fed him, changed the soiled bedding, gave him tablets and did everything, all the time looking worse and worse herself. My father was tenacious, a fighter to the death, of death. In the last few weeks he started occasionally talking about, but never quite admitting, that it was nearly all over. He was quite clear that, no matter how bad the pain, every moment of life was worth grabbing and hanging on to. For him any amount of pain was better than the alternative – not feeling anything at all ever again.

'I survived the ghettos and camps because of my will to live,' he said to me from his bed. 'Others just gave up. It was that and luck but maybe now my luck has run out.' This powerful desire to live was housed in a weaker and weaker body. Each day his voice lost strength; as it faded so did his life. It took him three years to die. In the end he had to go to hospital for the last week. The morphine he now needed to keep the pain dulled couldn't be given at home and my mother was no longer able to cope with looking after him and watching him die. At home still, on the day before he was going into hospital, my sister and I spent the day with my father. He dozed most of the time and said only two things distinctly and directly to us. 'It's the family, your mum, you, your children – that's what really matters and what made it all worth it for me. The rest was a waste of time, all for nothing.' The last thing he said to us was, 'Look after your Mummy.'

We visited the hospital every day, just sitting there. On what turned out to be his last evening he was like a crazy man trying, in his overwhelming weakness, to toss his head from side to side and move his hands. Too heavily sedated to recognise us, he rumbled and mumbled incoherently as if deliriously speaking in tongues. He wasn't even a person, and certainly not anyone we knew. It was horrible and the nurses shooed us out fairly soon. The next morning they rang: 'I'm sure you'll be pleased to know that your father went in his sleep last night, just like a lamb.' I didn't believe them - this is the same platitude they must trot out for everyone. There was never anything peaceful about him and he'd been the opposite of calm and serene when we'd left him.

To say that we are not a religious family is an under-statement. Although my father came from a religious family he had been a committed atheist since his teens. My mother seems never to have had any belief in God or religion to lose. I wondered if my father would have hung on for so long if he'd been religious. Surely it would dra-matically change your dying if you thought there was a mega purpose and plan and especially if, like the Mormons, you believed that you were going to join all the ever-youthful dead members of your family in Paradise. I can picture a Mormon blissfully lying there looking forward to being with her parents and her little son who'd died in a car accident. Such believers must be pleased to be called to Heaven, to the other world. I wonder how many people today die looking forward to their reward in Heaven? Being religious might have made my father less angry; may have taken away that stage of feeling it was unfair. But I can't imagine my father being religious. He became more tra-ditional as he got older, but never believed in any higher being.

It's not as if my father imagined he was immortal. As a member of a group that had already been chosen for death my father knew what awaited him. Perhaps he thought that as he'd outmanoeuvred it once, the same tricks would work again. His survival in the camps was not because of any long-term planning but taking his chances where he could find them, from moment to moment. This was the tactic he pursued, unsuccessfully this time, to fight his cancer.

Would things have been different if my parents had got to their three score years and ten? My father was 61 when he died and my mother 58, neither made it to living out their average life span. I don't think so. My father's death epitomised the way he was in life. Struggle was one of his favourite words. Despite his strong sense of history my father didn't finish what he called, 'my autobiography'. On the tape he describes his time in the concentration camp Maydanek and how one of the Kapos beat him with a thick fence post for the fun of it. 'He left me for dead,' Dad says, 'but I recovered. I think that's where my present sickness comes from. I've had problems with my stomach ever since that beating.' The story peters out. By this time his voice is slow, cracked and barely audible. The tape runs out mid-sentence … as if he never really stopped.

'Do you want me to go with you to see Mr Ansell?'

'No, Irwin will drive me. You don't need to take time off work. Anyway you've got the family to look after. Those lovely children, how are they, all healthy?'

I don't want to ring her when I get home from work. Any news is bad news. She won't ring me either if it's bad. I ring. 'He can't tell anything he says but I'm to have exploratory surgery soon at Prince Henry's.' If he thought there was nothing wrong she wouldn't be having exploratory surgery.

Between the time Mum went to see Ansell and the exploratory surgery a couple of weeks later I don't think either Mum or I slept much. It's when I started my addiction to detective stories. One a night, getting up to read after failing to fall asleep at about 1 a.m. and reading till 3 or so. It passed the time and at least for those few hours I managed to escape my thoughts and my dreams.

Each night the images were waiting to assail me.

My father-in-law in his hospital bed, crunched up in a foetal roll, looking like he'd been shrunken by headhunters to fit into a baby-size coffin. Me sitting at the hospital just crying for the pity of it all, that this is how we end up almost back to the size we started. He is sedated into unconsciousness and doesn't wake up again. Like my father he didn't want to let go a moment earlier than he had to. It was raining the day he was carried out on a stretcher to the ambulance for his final few days in hospital. 'It's good to feel the raindrops on my face,' he said.

The morgue where I went to identify my Aunty Rosa. I'd offered to do it blithely enough when the hospital had called and said this was necessary as Rosa had died after a successful eye operation, except that she never recovered from the anaesthetic. A curtain swishes open, cinema-style, to reveal the main attraction – a stiff, bluish-grey coloured waxwork, a skull without any hair. A monster and very dead. I'd no idea who it was but apparently this was my aunt. I won't be doing this again.

And the rolling and rerolling of the story of my father's death ending with his funeral at that bleak windswept cemetery. The rain soaked us as we listened to the heavy final thuds of sodden clods of mud landing on his coffin, echoing in my mind like a huge clock chiming *the end*.

I was the first one in to see my mother after the surgery. Before I could ask anything she said, 'It's what I thought. This time in the bowel. I'm not going to have any treatment and I don't want to suffer.' There was nothing for me to say, she'd already convinced me by her behaviour, even before they opened her up to have a look, that she had cancer. She's been thinking it all out for weeks. We didn't have to be cancer specialists to suspect it. Neither of us was surprised to be told that with this second bout of cancer there was no chance for her.

My sister came in and Mum repeated. 'It's bowel cancer.' Helen said, 'When will Ansell operate?' 'He can't operate - it's too late,' said my mother. 'You can have therapy can't you?' asked Helen. 'It's no use,' said Mum. Helen tried the usual reassurances and complacencies but Mum just looked at her and didn't answer.

After a silence I didn't know how to fill, Mum said, 'Tell Mr Ansell – you know they never listen to me – tell him that I'm not having any treatment. Go on Helen, tell him. He's nearby somewhere, try next door, as he's just been to see me. I don't want to argue, I'm too tired.'

This person giving firm, direct instructions was not the mother we'd got used to in the last ten years or so. She was more like the powerful mother of my childhood and adolescence. More recently Mum had become soft, self-effacing, the peace maker and peace lover. Today, from her high hospital bed, though she said she was tired, she was issuing edicts we had to carry out. Her voice was calm and sure, quite peremptory, unlike the woman who was too timid and embarrassed to attend any kind of leisure course in case she couldn't cope.

As soon as my sister had left to look for the doctor Mum said to me, 'You must do this for me. I don't want to suffer. Find something. Once I can't be at home anymore and can't look after myself I don't want to keep on living.'

I knew my mother was absolutely serious. She understood exactly what to expect, she'd been through it all with my father. She knew a lot better than I did what was at stake and had read the signs right away, well before she'd been to the doctor and been proved right.

The experience with my father had changed me too. This time I couldn't even be angry. The prospect of losing my mother was so frightening that I could hardly bear seeing her. Instead of enjoying her company over those last few months, for me every visit was a painful reminder of what wasn't going to be there any more very soon. I started thinking about being an orphan. There would be no one to care for me in that all-loving, all-forgiving way. The ache in me was almost overwhelming. It was waiting to consume me, to drag me into a depression I'd never be able to climb out of. Resisting going under took all my emotional effort. I had nothing left for worrying about others – not my sister, not Irwin, not my aunt. They'd have to look after themselves as I was concentrating on surviving myself. I got far too involved in various intractable problems at work, stupid factions and fights. Looking back I see that this was a way of avoiding dealing with my impending loss.

Irwin was my mother's live-in companion – maybe her lover. They had been living together since a year after my father died. They had in common a language and immigrant background, two grown children each, grandchildren, and the fact that both had nursed their partners through terminal cancers. Irwin obviously loved and was devoted to Mum but she wasn't giving all that much back. Maybe she felt more than she let on to us, her children, knowing that we would be angry if she showed that she loved anyone else but our father. I always think of him as 'Poor Irwin'. This was the second time for him – caring for his wife until she died, and now my mother.

A couple of months passed and we struggled along. Mum looked a bit frailer and was doing less. 'Come for a walk round the block with me,' she said, 'Irwin will play with the children.' I took her arm and we walked the familiar route we'd taken each summer evening after dinner for all the years I was growing up in this suburb. Most of the old pre-war Californian bungalows had been pulled down and replaced by clinker brick residences with two-car garages taking up most of their frontage. I knew I wouldn't be doing this walk for much longer.

'I'll never see any of my grandchildren grow up and marry. It's nearly time now,' Mum said. 'You must do it for me. I can't suffer any more. The doctor says that I should go into Bethlehem, a hospice. I won't go. What have you found out?'

'I don't see why you don't find out for yourself. You know your doctor really well; he's not a Catholic. There's no reason why I can do it any better than you.' My mother said very quietly, 'I want you to do this for me.' There was no way out for me, I couldn't refuse her.

'I haven't done anything yet,' I said. 'Are you sure?' I knew it was a stupid question but I had to say it. My mother said, 'I can't ask anybody else to do it.'

And so I rang a friend involved with the voluntary euthanasia movement who sent me some photocopied pages from Derek Humphry's book *Let Me Die Before I Wake*. 'You'll need to find a sympathetic doctor to get the prescriptions but the book tells you what you need and what works,' she said. I read the pages. In Chapter 2 there was a description of the way the author had assisted his first wife to die peacefully and when she chose to. This was what my mother wanted. The book's proselytising and somewhat self-satisfied tone did not appeal to me. Humphry seemed to have no qualms at all. I knew that I didn't want to help my mother to die. Would it be different with a partner than with a mother, the one who gave birth to me?

I put off ringing my general practitioner, who I thought would be sympathetic, for another couple of weeks. My mother said nothing when we saw each other but I knew she was waiting. I finally rang Ken and made an appointment for that day. The book said that I couldn't say I needed sleeping pills as I'd just get Mogadon or something else that wouldn't work. My mother had been taking one or two Mogadon a night for years already. So I had to be clear about what I wanted the pills for. I explained about my mother and how she didn't want to suffer. 'Are you sure she wants this?' Ken asked. 'She's very definite. The opposite to my father,' I said. 'Well I can't help you, you know it's illegal,' he said. I thought, what a bastard. 'But I can give you something to make her more comfortable,' and he nodded knowingly at me. 'This'll make it a bit easier for her,' he said, writing out two separate prescriptions. 'The prescriptions are in your name of course,' he said, 'I don't want any problems. They'll do the trick for what you want.'

This was the first time I felt angry about my situation. Why couldn't the bloody doctors do it, come over with an injection and that'd be it. Here was I, an amateur, forced to do their job and they wouldn't even provide me with efficient means. You'd think he could have given me a single strong pill or phial of something, instead of a prescription for two bottles of pills. It's a doctor's job to relieve suffering by medical means. I didn't have the expertise.

I rang Mum when I got home from the chemist, 'I've got the tablets. I'll bring them over tonight. You can take them whenever you want to.' 'No, you give them to me. I don't want to do it,' she said. 'But Mum, you're perfectly capable. I've got you the tablets, I've done what you asked me, take them when you're ready.' Mum said, 'I want you to do this for me. Please.' I couldn't refuse my mother's pleading. She didn't want to take responsibility for her own death even though that's what she'd chosen. I was to be the actor, the one who took responsibility.

Derek Humphry hadn't been reluctant but I was. It was partly the irony of the birth/death contrast but there was more to it. Some of it was resentment at being chosen for the role of assassin, being seen as the hard one in the family. Mum saw Helen as too soft and caring to be trusted to carry it through and my sister was happy for me to do it all. She knew what Mum had asked of me but hadn't offered to assist. We wanted Mum to have her way but, as well, we wanted to keep her with us as long as we could. There are powerful taboos at work – nobody wants to be a parent killer.

My major reluctance to do what my mother asked was that

I knew that, partly, she was doing it for me. She didn't want us to have to watch her die painfully and slowly, to burden me in the same way as Dad had her. She wanted to let us off the hook so that we didn't need to come and stay with her, feed her, take her to the toilet and watch her pain. Mum said that she didn't want to suffer but I knew that she also didn't want us to suffer with her. She didn't want to put us through what Dad had put her through. That was the big difference between them. My mother understood the demands her drawn-out dying would make on others as well as herself; my father only thought of himself.

There is nothing in their history to suggest that one was braver than the other. When it came to dealing with pain my mother, like most women, had always been a lot more stoical than my father. We used to laugh together about how hopeless men were when they were sick. 'It's just a cold and he's ready for the cemetery,' my mother said about my father. My mother wasn't afraid of pain. I'm sure that the suffering she feared was made up only to a small extent of physical pain. It was mostly the mental anguish at slowly disappearing with increasing bodily humiliations, and watching the pain and suffering reflected in all those she loved most. Knowing that she wanted the quick end as much for us as for her made it all nearly too much for me. I resisted being complicit in something that would be to my advantage.

That Sunday we had a family meeting, my mother, my sister and I. Mum seemed more content than she'd been for a long time. She now had a rest every morning and no longer went out at night but visitors came almost every evening to see her. Irwin did all the housework and shopping and looked after Mum's every want. She was still going out a bit in the day with him. They'd seen and enjoyed the play *Steaming* at a matinee. Mum said that she could only go about two hours before needing to rest or change her position and that she wasn't concentrating very well any more. The next weekend we were having a party in our garden with strawberries and cream and she was hoping to come. 'I'm lucky you know,' she said, 'I won an extra forty years in the lottery of life. My father was murdered when he wasn't even forty by rival pedlars in Rumania and the rest of my family were all killed by the Germans. Heniek and Fela, my brother and sister, were in their teens and even my mother was still a young woman. Cousins. Everyone. Me, I've got good children and grandchildren and I've had a wonderful life here in Australia. So maybe it's a bit early but look how happy we've been. You both married good people, you've got everything you need.'

For an excitable, noisy family we'd been very quiet these last few months. Sick people can't stand noise. There'd been none of the usual shouting and crying. If the children became noisy or started whooping, as children who have no idea of death do, we hustled them outside or took them home. We'd been dry-eyed, which for a five hankies per movie duo like my mother and me was unbelievable. But that day we made up for the drought. It was as if the three of us alone and knowing what we had to do had to let it all come out. We soon ran out of hankies and just let the tears flow.

My mother had it all planned. I was to organise the tablets. She'd let us know and would send Irwin away. 'Irwin,' she said, 'can't cope. He would get too upset. He's going to stay with Aunty Anka and they can stop each other from getting too nervous.' Helen and I would come over and stay the night to make sure that nothing went wrong. She'd give us enough notice so we could organise our families and, if need be, get time off work. Mum told us what she wanted to give people and had a list ready for us, mainly of jewellery for her nieces, and things her friends particularly liked.

The last time she left the house was to come to our party. It was a glorious December day. Dressed in her best, make-up on and hair done, she was looking good despite the hollow cheeks and too-thin arms. The sun shone gently on her in the deckchair where Irwin had placed her and from which she didn't move for the two hours she was there. It's very hard for people to talk naturally or normally to someone who's dying. People were awkward. They couldn't say, 'How long have you got to go?' like they would with a pregnant woman. And it's very hard to make small talk to someone who you know is facing extinction. People came up, chatted for a while as if to pay their last respects. At one stage they were even lined up. When Irwin took her home and I walked her out to the car I could see that she was exhausted. 'Don't worry,' she said, 'I'm not in pain. I enjoyed the party. Very interesting to see how all those wild girlfriends of yours have settled into middle age.'

Mum was now spending most of each day in bed, still managing to go to the toilet on her own. She was asking visitors to come one at a time and not stay for too long as she found them tiring.

In January I was staying down at the beach and driving up to see Mum every couple of days. Helen, who lived near Mum, popped in every day. I spoke to Mum on the phone every day. One Friday evening, just after we'd eaten, she rang. 'The doctor says I must go into Bethlehem on Monday, after the weekend. I'm not going. I want you to come and stay tomorrow night.' 'Okay, I'll be there and we'll all have a meal together,' I said. 'I'll ring and tell Helen.'

It was only about six months since she'd come back from Hawaii, I thought. The stress and anxiety that I had been holding down by skating over what was happening threatened to rise up and engulf me. Tomorrow I would have no mother. It struck me how incredibly selfish my anxiety was – it was all about my loss. I don't know what I would have done if the choice to turn off the life-supports or whatever had been mine, if my mother had not been conscious enough to make her own views known. She had never spoken about euthanasia or even thought about it as far as I knew until her bowel cancer was diagnosed. I can't recall anything at all she said prior to that which would have given me any clue as to what she'd want. Maybe I'd have thought she would be like my father, or that she'd want to go on with her usual stoicism. With my selfishness I might have thought she'd want to live as long as possible no matter at what cost so she could still see us, her children and grandchildren. Calculating benefit to myself would have been impossible – the pleasure of having her with me, against the anguish of having to watch her die like my father did, become a non-person.

Driving along the Nepean Highway I had the radio on full blast trying to blot out what came next. But every song, no matter how banal, seemed specially chosen to break me down. I cried for the forty minutes it took me to get there, wiping my face with eau de cologne to remove all traces before I went in.

Irwin was waiting for me looking as miserable as a human being could be. As usual he made me feel guilty that I hadn't been the one looking after her, guilty that I hadn't been nicer to him, and guilty because I felt he disapproved of what I was going to do. 'She's settled down now,' he said. 'I'll be going to Anka's. I'll keep Anka company for dinner.' Now that I thought about it I was surprised that he was going to my Aunt's place rather than to stay with his children. I said this to Helen when she arrived, arms laden with food. Helen said, 'It's for security. We can't let everybody know because it's not legal. That's why Mum's being a bit cagey and not saying anything right out.' 'She's pretty straight about what she wants from me,' I said.

Helen cooked schnitzel with baby potatoes and coleslaw, Mum's favourites. We sat on her bed with our plates on our knees. Mum looked a little tired and weak but that's all. She ate a bit of everything to please us. I'd brought a bottle of wine because I wanted to make things festive but also because it said in *Let Me Die Before I Wake* that alcohol makes the pills more potent. Mum sipped a mouthful of wine but we could see that she liked it as little as ever. A light meal also helps the ingestion of drugs.

My mother went over her funeral arrangements again and we told her what we'd been doing. No one looking in at us would have thought anything of moment was happening, just a family meal in the bedroom. For me everything was charged with emotion, making itself felt in my chest and stomach as weight and constriction. My mind was cool, iced, detached from the turmoil going on in the body underneath. I knew what she wanted me to do and I was going to do it.

I went to my handbag and got out the two bottles of capsules, fifty in each bottle, one bottle of Amytal and one of Nembutal. From the book I had learned that to make them more effective it was better to open them and mix the powder with water or some other liquid. This took me quite a while. I concentrated carefully so as not to lose any powder. I made us all a cup of tea and went back into the bedroom where Mum and my sister were waiting. 'This'll be very bitter, Mum. I didn't know whether I should mix sugar in it or if that'll have some effect on the tablets.' 'It'll be fine without sugar. You know I've never taken sugar in anything,' she said. I mixed a bit of tea into the powder in the cup and gave it to Mum to drink as Helen and I sat watching.

Her face twisted at the bitterness of the taste as she swallowed. 'Could I have a teaspoon to scrape the rest of it out?' she asked. When she'd finished we all had a cup of tea together. Mum was already getting drowsy and only just managed to say, 'Thankyou for doing this for me ... ' before falling asleep. I grabbbed the cup before the rest of the tea spilt. Her breathing was loud and laboured. I tucked her arms in under her eiderdown, straightened up her pillow, and, with Helen, left the bedroom.

I felt calmer, more relaxed, knowing I'd been able to go through with what she wanted. Helen and I talked and read a bit, going in to see Mum every twenty minutes or so. She didn't move but her breathing became louder, more rasping, almost painful. By midnight there had been no change and I was getting worried. My sister looked absolutely exhausted so I sent her off to have a sleep. 'Are you sure?' she said. 'Will you be all right?' 'I haven't been sleeping all that much lately so I'm used to it,' I said. 'I'll wake you if anything happens.'

There was nothing escapist to watch on TV so I read some more of Blanche d'Alpuget's biography of Bob Hawke, not taking much of it in and not caring. I couldn't sit in the room with Mum because of the awful racket she was making. Humphry had said nothing to prepare me for this terrible noise. Her breathing sounded as if it was coming through great internal pain, though her face remained composed. My mother was neither smiling nor frowning but looked settled. This was not the beautiful calm experience Humphry had described. I felt the same resentment I'd had towards the natural childbirth teacher who'd conned me into believing that contractions were like ripples in a pond and that a painfree birth could be achieved by learning the right breathing techniques. I hadn't said anything to my sister because I didn't want to get her worried as well. Organising the tablets had been my responsibility. Why hadn't anything happened yet? She'd taken the stuff at 9 p.m. and it was now 3 a.m. Maybe it wasn't going to work and she'd soon wake up from a deep sleep.

I went in again several times. The third time, at 3.40, I raised her left arm. It fell back lifelessly but the booming breathing still continued. I lifted her eyelids; her eyes stared at me accusingly. Had I failed to carry out her wishes? I should have checked the dosage and the content of those tablets more scientifically instead of just accepting them from the doctor. Maybe they were the wrong thing. Perhaps all that medication my mother took for her various ailments made her less susceptible.

Sitting at the kitchen table I realised how quickly the night was disappearing. Helen would wake and Irwin would come home. We couldn't do this a second time, it was hard enough doing it once.

Light was starting to come in under the venetian blinds. I went in again and looked at Mum. There was no change. She looked asleep but the noise of a two-stroke engine was coming from her. I picked up the pillow beside her, the one that had been my father's, and pressed it down gently on her face. The noise abated. I pressed it more firmly over her nose and mouth until she made no sound. I took the pillow away and kissed her. Then I replaced the pillow and checked that she wasn't breathing. My mother was dead.

I'm not sure how long I sat on the bed, maybe for an hour. I was in a kind of trance at what I'd done. It's not that I felt guilty or bad or that I'd done wrong but I understood the magnitude of what I'd done.

I woke my sister, 'She died,' I said. Helen went in to see her and we both kissed her and tucked her in yet again. These small protective, affectionate gestures just continue whether the person appreciates them or not.

Helen did all the organising after that and I went to bed. I fell asleep immediately. By the time I awoke Irwin was back and the funeral organised. Mum's general practitioner, Mr Graham, had been and according to Helen said, 'She was going into the Bethlehem on Monday so maybe it's all for the best.' He signed the death certificate and put 'heart failure' as the cause of death.

We waited with a sobbing Irwin who probably thought Helen and I were made of stone until the Jewish funeral company came to take her body away. The funeral would be tomorrow. By the time the Chevra Kadisha took her away she was a corpse not a person, and as her stiff pasty-grey mask went past me I too broke down – my mother was gone.

I told my husband when I got home that night what I'd

done. He looked at me in a strange way, suggesting surprise and some awe at my action, not criticism. 'I didn't plan it. I still don't know how I did it. I just knew I had to. I couldn't let her wake up, she would not have forgiven me.'

Until early this year no one else knew. On the tenth anniversary I told my sister. I thought it was time she knew. Helen's reaction was strangely like my husband's. Shock but not shock-horror, more surprise that I had the strength to do this.

Writing about what happened has been more difficult and painful than I'd imagined. I felt the same weight and constriction when I wrote about my mother's last night as I felt on the night itself. I've never been sorry or guilty about what I did. I've never had an abortion but I imagine that if I'd had to have one this is what I would feel like. I did something I had to do, I did the right thing, the decent and correct thing, but it was an awful thing to have to do and I hope that I never have to do it again.

NOTE

1. Names and other details have been altered to protect the anonymity of those concerned.

There Has to Be
a More Humane Way

The events I am going to recount happened only relatively recently. Writing about them will be extremely painful. But no matter how painful this process will be, I am going to tell the story of my husband's death. I am doing this because I firmly believe that Charles should not have died the way he did. There has to be a more humane way. I very much hope that my narrative will help us find that way.

Charles and I had been married for over ten years. We were both in the medical profession – he as a palliative care registered nurse and I as a medical practitioner.

As health care professionals we had both witnessed much tragedy and suffering. Early in our relationship we had therefore made a pact that if some accident or medical condition deprived one of us of our dignity or quality of life, we would not allow the other to suffer. Our trust in one another in this matter was complete. This attitude

The author is a medical practitioner, but not currently working in her profession. Shaken by her husband's death and disillusioned by the direction the medical profession is taking as a whole, she is planning to enter the business world. She believes that she cannot be part of a profession that does not adequately respect the human rights of patients. She is an active member of a Voluntary Euthanasia Society.

stemmed from our belief that each individual has, firstly, the right to determine what quality of life is acceptable to her or him and, secondly, the inherent right to choose when to die should that quality irredeemably be lost.

We were both in our mid-thirties with small children when my husband was diagnosed as having an incurable disease. There was no treatment and a terrible uncertainty: the condition would result in Charles lapsing into a vegetative state - either suddenly or progressively. We sought many expert medical opinions and made extensive enquiries as to future prospects of treatment, unfortunately to no avail. Once these opinions had confirmed the hopelessness of the situation, we had to consider our options.

Charles's present quality of life was normal, in the physical sense. He was working full time, driving a car, and everything would have seemed fine to the medically untrained eye. Nonetheless, we knew that his memory had deteriorated markedly and that he was having difficulty controlling the movements in his right arm and leg. The symptoms were, however, only noticeable to those very close to him.

As I've mentioned, the condition Charles was suffering from was unpredictable. It had several ways of behaving – there could either be a sudden exarcerbation (resulting in an instantaneous vegetative state), or the condition might progress more slowly, in stages, to the same vegetative state. No one was able to predict which course it would follow.

This posed a particularly difficult problem for us. If Charles were to take his own life, he had to be able to carry out that procedure himself, in order not to implicate me. But that was just the problem. We did not know how much time we had left. If Charles did not take his life soon, he might miss the opportunity of doing so. On the other hand, if he were to take his life now, while still able to do so, how much good quality life would he be sacrificing?

Choosing when to end his life was not a legally available

option. It was this very fact that made us so angry with society – in effect society was robbing Charles and our family of an unknown quantity of good life together.

Charles decided, with my full support, that he could not wait and risk lapsing into a vegetative state. He was young and healthy and would, in all likelihood, have survived for many years, unable to move, to communicate, and to recognise me or the children. Charles loved his family too much and had too much dignity as a man to risk such a situation.

Charles used the weeks following his diagnosis to finalise his affairs. Six weeks later, we, as a couple, decided on a date when he would end his life. Throughout this entire process we made all decisions together. We also began to prepare the children for their father's impending death. This was the most upsetting and emotionally taxing thing we had to do. Only weeks before, our children had lost an immediate family member to whom they were very close. It was also extremely difficult to explain to the children *why* their father was going to die, as the symptoms of his disease were only visible to a very discerning medical eye. From the children's viewpoint, their father looked healthy. This was quite different from the relative, who had died recently, after having deteriorated quite noticeably over many months.

Before deciding on a date, we had already decided on the medication to be used and had been able to obtain it in sufficient quantities. Charles decided to ingest a far greater quantity than was considered to be the fatal dose to make certain nothing would go wrong.

During the final day, we carried out the normal family routine, both quite detached from what was to take place that evening. We were totally resolved and of one mind with respect to our decision.

Charles wrote a suicide note stating the reasons why he was going to take his life. To ensure that I would not be implicated in any way, Charles also stated clearly that he alone had made the decision to end his life, and that he alone would carry it out.

That evening when the children were asleep we spent our last hours together before Charles swallowed the tablets. We both took a sleeping tablet and went to bed. We had both researched the toxic and fatal effects of this drug, and read about the expected manner of death. One can never be quite certain how a particular drug will affect an individual, but what happened during that night was not what either of us had expected or read about in the relevant literature.

I was unable to sleep even with the strong sleeping tablet I had taken. Charles, on the other hand, had soon fallen into a semiconscious state. The ensuing hours were the most emotionally traumatic of my life. Charles convulsed violently for eight hours. By 5 a.m. I was in a state of panic as I came to the realisation that this medication was, in all likelihood, not going to prove fatal. According to the pharmaceutical and toxicological information we had gathered, death should have occurred within two to three hours. Many hours later, Charles was still alive. He was unconscious but very restless, and I was fully aware of the possible permanent damage of surviving such an overdose.

Between 5 and 6 a.m. I was so emotionally and physically drained that I cannot find the words to describe the terror I felt.

I knew I had to make a decision: the children would be waking very soon. I left the bedroom and was shaking quite uncontrollably. The only way I can describe what happened next is that I completely 'switched off' emotionally and became exclusively rational. I knew what had to be done.

I went back up to the bedroom and placed a pillow over my husband's head and lay on it for over ten minutes, until there was no breathing and no pulse. I realised that I was taking a risk because the manner of death might be detected, but there was no choice. I had to complete the process my husband had begun.

No one should have to experience what happened that morning and the preceding night.

There is a part of me I can never share with another human being. I could do what was necessary that morning only because we, as a couple, had decided that it was best, under the circumstances. There simply were no other options available to us. If we could have ensured that Charles would not be kept alive indefinitely in a vegetative state, and if euthanasia had been available to him when he no longer considered his quality of life satisfactory, I would have been able to have the loving support of my family around me when he died. Also, Charles might have been with us for some weeks or months yet. In any case, I am thankful that it is unlikely that he was aware of my suffering.

In one way, we were luckier than others who find themselves in a similar situation. Because we were both in the medical profession, the drugs we needed were freely available. However, even though we had done a lot of research, things did not go according to plan.

I am angry about three issues – all of them related to the fact that voluntary euthanasia is still unlawful. First, owing to the unpredictability of Charles's medical condition and the threat of him lapsing into a vegetative state, he and his family had to forfeit an unknown quantity of 'quality life'. Charles had to end his life earlier than he would have if voluntary euthanasia had been lawful. Second, we were forced to use an uncertain method of suicide. Had voluntary euthanasia been legal, Charles's death would not only have been certain, but also much quicker and less traumatic. Third, if voluntary euthanasia had been lawful, I, as his wife, would have been spared the absolute horror of that evening and the following morning. I would not have been alone.

Charles and I believed that each person must decide what

quality of life is acceptable to her or him. Nobody else can, or should, have the right to make that decision. Once a person has reached that decision, then, we believed, it should be lawful to help that person to end her or his life in a way that is certain and comfortable. Charles, of course, is dead now. But I still hold these views - and more strongly than ever. Charles should not have died the way he did. There must be a better way.

Anonymous

Death Without Dignity

I feel compelled to tell the sad story of the way my dear partner died and of the trauma and heartache he and his loved ones suffered in the process.

Geoffrey was my partner, and he would have wished the publication of this account of the manner of his death if it could be used to further the cause of legalising medically assisted dying in this country. We so desperately desired it for him then.

Geoffrey and I met and became partners in our middle years. Our respective children had grown up, and we found much joy together sharing similar interests and philosophies.

Neither of us was religious. We took the view that humans are responsible for their own destinies and must face their problems with their own moral and intellectual resources, and we did not believe in an 'afterlife'. However, we were both convinced that hopelessly ill

The author is a nurse, a profession she loves. She was born overseas, but has lived in Australia for the past thirty years. Before meeting Geoffrey, she had been married and raised a family. After Geoffrey's death, the author returned to work. Her happy memories of her eight-year relationship with her partner Geoffrey, and her work, have sustained her. Her continuing involvement in the committees in which both were active, and family commitment to an aged parent ensure that her time is well occupied.

49

people should have the legal option of active medical help in dying, on serious request.

As a young man Geoffrey had witnessed his father dying slowly of a terminal cancer at home. The poor man had spent many hours hiccoughing before he eventually died. Geoffrey was appalled by his father's misery and decided that he would not wish to continue living under similar circumstances, and would seek medical intervention to end his life before that stage was reached.

As a nurse, I had also seen many instances of prolonged suffering ending in certain death, and had cause to remember the time when I and my colleagues assisted an old woman in her eighties to die. This patient was privileged in that her daughter was an anaesthetist at the hospital, and was able to supervise her medication. The woman seemed desperate to die and wanted to be put out of her misery. She was suffering from a debilitating chronic disease and was bedridden and in constant discomfort. She asked all who tended her to help her to die.

Morphine injections were ordered and mercifully death resulted three days later. One of the nurses refused to give the injections. She was a Roman Catholic but despite her moral or religious objections, she did not report the matter.

This happened many years ago in an overseas hospital, but the incident helped to positively shape my views on voluntary euthanasia. We were practising euthanasia, under medical direction, even if nobody called it that, and even though it took three long days for death to occur.

Geoffrey and I were enjoying life. He had retired early, was kept stimulated and very active on three committees, and was pursuing various other interests as well. I was working full time with retirement in sight, and we were anticipating a happy future.

I am so thankful for those eight happy years with a wonderful person because it was soon to end tragically.

The first inkling of trouble came when Geoffrey discovered a lump in his abdomen. He took two weeks to tell me about it. I urged him to seek medical advice, fearing the worst and remembering the story of his father's illness.

It was not long before the worst was confirmed: an inoperable cancer similar to that from which his father had died, and at the same time of life. After a bowel bypass operation, a prognosis of between four and eighteen months was given. We were devastated.

It was suggested to try chemotherapy, which Geoffrey was told by a specialist would give him a one in four chance of remission. Being the positive, optimistic person he was, he accepted this and became convinced that he could beat the disease. In the meantime, I had taken extended leave from my employment and moved in with Geoffrey to care for him as he had developed a severe wound infection after the operation. Despite this, he remained positive and cheerful as chemotherapy had commenced and he was tolerating it well.

Geoffrey decided he would talk to the doctors treating him about medically assisted death, in the hope of finding someone who would help him when he was ready to die. We did eventually find a compassionate doctor who said he would order morphine to induce coma whenever Geoffrey decided that he had had enough, and would let nature take its course with pneumonia causing death.

We were happy to accept this as we realised that it would be impossible to obtain a lethal dose. No doctor would be willing to break the law and risk prosecution to bring about a quick death, particularly for an unknown patient.

We then put the whole matter to the back of our minds as Geoffrey was feeling better and was still positive that he would beat the disease anyway. We managed to have some lovely holidays together and with friends, after which I returned to work. Geoffrey was still coping well with the chemotherapy and, although he had to forgo his more active pursuits, he managed to enjoy life.

This continued for fourteen months. Chemotherapy was then stopped; scans had shown no increase in the size of the tumour and it was thought that Geoffrey was in remission.

After four months, however, Geoffrey's condition started to deteriorate. His surgeon was consulted and another bowel bypass operation confirmed that life was only likely for a few more months. Geoffrey, though, was not giving up and sought more chemotherapy from his specialist. Again he was told that there was still a one in four chance of remission, and so resumed chemotherapy. I was fortunate enough to be able to take leave without pay to care for him.

Geoffrey was unable to tolerate the chemotherapy in his weakened state, needing daily enemas and feeling very unwell. Somehow, with help from our friends we managed to sell his house and move to mine to be near our compassionate doctor. Geoffrey was loath to leave his garden.

Incredibly, after a few weeks his condition improved. Chemotherapy was recommenced. By this time four-hourly morphine and antidepressants were being administered. He was able to enjoy the company of old friends from interstate and even to work in the garden.

Eleven months after the second operation his condition deteriorated once more. He was losing control of his urinary function and becoming very anxious about his state of health. The Home Nursing Service was consulted and Geoffrey was persuaded to use a syringe-driver (a battery-operated syringe which he could control to maintain a steady dose of morphine in his body). His specialist ordered another scan and poor Geoffrey willingly underwent great discomfort to have confirmed what to me was obvious: that further growths were present.

Geoffrey at last accepted that his condition was terminal

and nothing further could be done. He talked to his children about his plans to die very soon and although they were sorrowful they understood how he felt. We decided to have a party and invite all his many friends to say goodbye, followed by a family gathering the next day. He enjoyed the party in his bedroom and the following day sadly farewelled his devoted family.

Our doctor was in full agreement with Geoffrey's decision that the time had come, feeling it was medically appropriate. He ordered a much increased dose of morphine and other sedatives to be commenced when the nurses next visited in the evening.

We made our farewells tearfully, thanked each other for the joys we had shared, and kissed. Geoffrey then seemed at peace with himself and I was beginning to feel relieved that soon his suffering would be over. The nursing staff came to begin treatment and soon Geoffrey was asleep.

I was frequently at his bedside that night, giving him further shots of the medication by pressing the controls of the syringe-driver. He was sleeping heavily. He needed changing once and I was so glad he was unaware as he would have been mortified. In the morning I was assisted to bathe him. He was still deeply asleep and all was going according to plan.

But it was not to be. Passing his open door later that morning, I was horrified to see Geoffrey awake, confused and struggling to sit up. He had slept for sixteen hours.

Again our doctor came and suggested using a stronger form of morphine and other sedatives. Geoffrey agreed and the new treatment was commenced.

The nurses were calling regularly to supervise the syringe-driver and to check the drugs. I was alway uneasy about their vigilance in recording the amount used as I never dared to discuss voluntary euthanasia, fearing they would guess at our intentions.

In spite of the heavier medication, Geoffrey was able to

sleep only for short periods. I was by this time mentally and physically exhausted and unable to think objectively. We both knew that his release would not come this way. He was in great mental and physical discomfort, constantly worried about urination and needing enemas, but would only accept sips of water.

Finally, in absolute desperation, I remembered a very good friend of Geoffrey's who had always given sound advice in troubled times. I called him and thankfully he came. Geoffrey was able to tell him how much he wanted to die but could not. We discussed methods of dying again, as we had in the past, and remembered the plastic bag method. Here was our answer to bring about peace for Geoffrey.

Months ago, Geoffrey had placed a bag of suitable size in a convenient drawer and now he directed me to it. I knew I had to take the responsibility, and I realised the best time would be later that day after the visit of different nurses on the next shift. We thanked our visitor and sadly said goodbye.

We then made our plan. After the nurses left later that day I fed my poor darling a handful of sleeping pills with a glass of warm milk and water. He swallowed those pills so eagerly. We kissed again and he was soon fast asleep and snoring.

Three hours later, Geoffrey was still snoring and I decided, sick in the stomach, that I had to do the deed. I knew I could not fail him now. I placed the bag over his relaxed head and secured the ends with a towel. It took ten minutes for his breathing to become laboured, and then the sides of the bag were drawn in with every gasping breath. His poor emaciated body hardly moved during this time. At the end of twenty minutes, breathing had ceased and I could not feel a pulse.

I removed the bag and towel, folded Geoffrey's hands on his chest and closed his eyes. I turned off the syringe-driver and, in a daze, left the room.

Then I realised that his agony as well as mine was over, and poured myself a stiff brandy. I managed to ring our doctor, who said he would visit first thing in the morning, and then I slept for a while.

In the morning a dear friend came to help with the duties that the bereaved have to perform and our doctor arrived. He was relieved that Geoffrey had died and I did not tell him how. He wrote 'cardio-pulmonary failure' on the death certificate.

It is now several years since this tragic episode in my life, the memory of which I shall never erase. I am angry that we were robbed of a decent parting. We had to endure in the midst of our grief a nightmare of repeated goodbyes and a death that need not have been so uselessly harrowing. We had to endure this because of our outdated laws and for no other reason. This I cannot accept, and I will never give up the fight for more sensible laws governing the way we die.

Mary Mortimer

New Year's Eve

Fourteen years ago, I broke the law. Technically, I may have committed murder. Apart from parking offences and civil disobedience – actions against the Vietnam War, against apartheid, in favour of a woman's right to choose, to name a few – I am not aware that I have broken the law before or since. In helping my first husband to take his life when it had become intolerable to him, the law says I committed a terrible act. For me, a much more terrible act would have been to watch him deteriorate physically and mentally, to know how unbearable this was for him, and to do nothing. I have never regretted that act. I have remained silent about it for many years, even to my children, for fear of criminal prosecution. But the debate has moved on, and there is widespread opinion that to legalise voluntary euthanasia

Mary Mortimer, teacher, author, librarian and feminist, was born in Tamworth, NSW, in 1944. Since graduating from Sydney University she has had a long career in education. Her interest in politics and social issues is reflected in her book, *Boys Do, Girls Are* (1979), and many articles on the sex stereotyping of children.

A past National Convenor of the National Foundation for Australian Women, Mary continues to work for women's groups, and now teaches Library Studies at the Canberra Institute of Technology. In 1991 she published *When Your Partner Dies.* Mary has two children and remarried in 1992.

would be just and humane. I hope that stories like mine will encourage serious, caring people to support this change.

Rex Mortimer was a highly intelligent and thoughtful maverick. He had a fine sense of fun and found status and pomp ridiculous. He was committed to understanding and improving human conditions. He was much older than me, and had clear ideas about what he wanted to do with his life, yet he was open to my ideas and different approaches to living. Sometimes reluctantly at first, he cheerfully adjusted to each new venture in our lives. He was a devoted father, who had wanted children for a long time (he was 44 when Michael was born), and fully shared the responsibilities of parenting.

He was 53 when cancer was diagnosed. He was Associate Professor of Government and Dean of Economics at Sydney University. He had published many books and articles, and was highly regarded as a creative thinker, a powerful teacher and a humane administrator. He was the proud father of Michael and Rachel, aged 9 and 7, and my loving husband.

His cancer began in the lung, and travelled quickly to his spine and then to his brain. He endured considerable, sometimes extreme, physical pain, though this could largely be controlled by drugs. However, long before anyone else was aware of it, he noticed that his speech was beginning to slur, and that he could not always put his tongue to the precise word he wanted. Of course this frustrated and worried him. Soon he felt unable to continue teaching, as he began to doubt that his brain was still functioning properly.

He greatly feared losing his dignity, indeed 'losing his mind'. He was afraid that the end of his life would be humiliating, and that our memory of him would be of a sick, incapable, irrational 'patient' rather than the full human being he was in our lives.

So we discussed how his life could be ended when *he* chose, when he felt it had become meaningless and abhorrent to him. We shared the attitude that life is more than existence, not simply the basic functioning of bodily organs. We agreed that, just as we had always aimed to exercise as much control as we could over our lives, we desired to have the same control over the way we died.

An understanding doctor visited us at home, and talked about quality of life, and about not prolonging life without meaning. He said he agreed with our view, and would be there to help us when Rex felt the time had come. But because of the (then) illegality of suicide and the (continuing) illegality of assisting suicide, he was taking a genuine risk encouraging us to think in this way. He would certainly have lost his right to practise medicine, and could have faced criminal prosecution and up to ten years in gaol for 'assisting, aiding and abetting, or counselling a person to commit suicide'. So he seemed to us to talk in riddles, and we tried not to be insensitive by asking direct questions. Little was actually said, though much was hinted at. We remained anxious and uncertain about what would eventually happen.

Rex hung on bravely, and even came home for Christmas which, though painfully sad for us, seemed to comfort the children. By Boxing Day, though, he wished his life to end quickly, while he still felt a whole person, to himself and to his family. We decided that it would be easier for me, and especially for the children, if he died in hospital, as I was not confident about coping with the additional responsibility on my own. We also thought that if he needed to take his own life, fewer questions would be asked if he was in hospital. So back he went, and I followed the ambulance, knowing that this was the beginning of his final journey out of our lives.

Within a few days, having been taken off all medication at his own request, but facing the prospect of lingering for at least some weeks, he took a large dose of sleeping pills. We said our final farewells, I sat with him until he dozed off, and went home to await the inevitable call from the hospital to tell me he had died in his sleep.

Except that it didn't come. After a long sleepless night I phoned the ward, to be told by a cheerful sister that he had slept well and was eating his breakfast! By the time I reached the hospital he was distraught, confused and slightly incoherent, but absolutely clear that he shouldn't still be here.

We held hands through the day. I didn't let the children visit, as they had already seen him for the last time as he wanted to be remembered. That day, New Year's Eve, I knew I had to try again, as I could stand his anguish and indignity no longer. I phoned the doctor from the hospital, talking as obscurely as I could about the situation. He told me he would leave a prescription for sleeping pills at an all-night chemist. It was for twenty tablets, and I should give nineteen to Rex, and keep one for myself (did he really think I could then go home and sleep?).

In the middle of the evening I left Rex dozing, muttered something to the nurse about having to go out for a while and being back later, and made my furtive trip to the chemist's. Even this was not straightforward: the pills were only half the strength the doctor said they would be, so did Rex need twice as many? Who could I ask? I couldn't contact the doctor again. Here I was in a large teaching hospital, surrounded by highly skilled staff who must have known the answer, but I couldn't ask anyone, since we were breaking the law. Rex wanted his life to end, and as he now needed help and I loved him, I was committed to performing this final act of loving kindness for him. Yet we were on our own. Fourteen years later, I still feel the rage and despair of being abandoned in our urgent need. That a beloved partner has to die is enough to bear; that enabling him or her to die with dignity should be accompanied by such terror and helplessness is an outrage in a society that considers itself civilised or caring.

I waited until the last nursing round, when I took his regular pills from the nurse and offered to give them to him when he woke. I was terrified: of being discovered, of too small a dose and failing again, of too large a dose and making him sick. By now he was too confused to take the pills by himself, so I fed them to him. Fearful of failing again, but not knowing the appropriate dose, I gave him as many pills as he could swallow. I kissed him, and then read him 'to sleep'. I was terrified, but determined to see it through.

I don't know when he died. I have no medical training and had no experience of death. Was the breathing noise that seemed to come from his chest the 'death rattle' I had heard of, but didn't understand? Was the pulse I felt for in his throat his or mine? I tried putting a mirror to his lips – was I doing it properly? How would I know?

So I sat, heart in mouth, holding his hand (still warm), reading. Until the midnight hospital round, and a sister who *did* know how to tell felt for his pulse and found nothing.

Even then it was not over. I was expelled from the room while a doctor was summoned. Would they try to revive him? Pump his stomach? Was it finished for him yet? I burst into the room, begging them to let him be; he wanted to die. He had died and they didn't try to resuscitate him; for Rex it was finally over.

As for me, I still had to engage with a young and inexperienced doctor. I refused a post-mortem, and became angry when he tried to persuade me to sign the papers. 'Standard hospital procedure', he said. Frightened as I was, I told him what I thought of standard hospital procedures, where routine seemed too often to take precedence over the real need of patients. 'I put up with all this for Rex's sake,' I said through clenched teeth, 'but now that he's gone I don't have to put up with it any longer!' Of course he was not to know what an angonising experience I had just had, and how terrified I still was. Would they discover the overdose if a post-mortem was performed? Could they find out anyway? I had no idea.

Eventually I was taken home by my sister- and brother-in-law, but I couldn't tell them either; how did I know what their reactions would be? So I lay awake all night, not yet able to grieve, waiting instead for the police to knock on my door and arrest me for murder.

Opponents of voluntary euthanasia say that decisions of life and death belong to God, not to men and women. They offer simplistic alternatives : patients can refuse medical treatment; palliative care eliminates pain; some even support the right of patients to take their own lives, but urge that no one else, including doctors, be involved!

None of these alternatives would have met Rex's needs.

Neither of us believed in God. Religious objections to moral acts must be considered by members of each particular faith. They should not be regarded as a valid basis for civil law. Our society has a very wide range of religious persuasions, and particular faiths must deal with moral issues within their own communities. Indeed, not all members of a particular religion agree about voluntary euthanasia. A friend was heartened by her Anglican priest's sermon on the subject. He concluded that if we wish to become a more humane society we will have to rethink our attitude to people dying in pain and suffering, when we have the means to help them to die with dignity.

Refusal of further life-sustaining medication will shorten life, but leaves the patient at the mercy of the natural deterioration of his or her body. This is particularly unsatisfactory if the illness is in the brain; in some cases the body may be quite strong, and take a long time to cease functioning. In this situation, a day is a long time, and the end can take weeks or even months.

Having asked to be taken off the medication which was keeping him alive, Rex could have lived through many weeks of diminishing mental capacity, which he could not bear. The months of his illness, and especially the last confused day of his life, when he rambled in and out of sensible communication with me, haunted me for months after his death, and I found it hard to remember him as a complete, competent person.

Palliative care can now effectively eliminate pain for many patients, and is a wonderfully humane development in medical practice. There are many patients with terminal illnesses for whom this is a good solution. A close friend died of leukaemia. Palliative care – in her case wearing a syringe-driver which administered small doses of morphine at regular intervals day and night – kept her pain at bay. She was able to come to terms with dying, and achieved a remarkable acceptance of her approaching death.

There are nevertheless many patients for whom this is not a solution.

My father had emphysema. The problem was not pain, but a decreasing store of energy. He had always been active, physically and mentally. He maintained his mental agility, and did everything he could to continue to live a full life. He read, wrote his family's history, engaged in philosophical conversation with all the clerics and intellectuals in the small country town where he lived. But he could no longer go walking, work in the garden, even eventually look after himself. After many months of physical deterioration, he was ready to die. He had tied off all the loose ends of his life and it held no more for him. He asked me to help him, but I could do nothing. A doctor could have. It was a frustrating end to a life he had enjoyed and over which he had exercised considerable control.

Illness affecting the brain reduces a person's mental capacity. Where the person is aware of this, it is humiliating; in any case most of us do not wish to become helpless, dependent or incapable of adult relationships with our friends and family.

For Rex this was of special concern. He had lived by his intelligence and wit, as a journalist and academic. His writing and public speaking were much admired; he was sparkling company. The effects of cancer on his brain horrified him. He could not countenance becoming incoherent or unable to think clearly. He was equally appalled that his family, in particular his small children, might remember him as less than the wonderful husband and father he had been. It was vital for him to end his life while he still exercised some control.

Some believe it is acceptable for people to take their own lives but not for others, especially medical specialists, to help them. This is fanciful, since it ignores the reality of terminal illness. Fairly soon after diagnosis many people are clear about how they wish their lives to end. This does not mean they are ready to die. If they had the choice, they would choose to live their lives fully for as long as possible. When life no longer held enough meaning for them, they would wish to end it. Unfortunately this is often when they lose their independence. This is precisely why they need assistance, having made their wishes clearly known while they were still competent to do so.

Rex was fairly sure that he would have this choice when the time came, although we could not be altogether confident, since what we planned was against the law.

He took the first overdose of sleeping pills while he was still fully conscious of what he was doing. But it failed to end his life since his body had built up a tolerance to drugs much greater than that of a 'normal' person. He needed assistance to take the second overdose, since his condition had deteriorated. There can be no doubt, however, that this is what he wanted, and that my action was fully in accordance with his wishes.

How could any lay person, patient or family member, know enough about drug tolerance and bodily function to assess the likely effects of any drug in this situation? It is clearly necessary for doctors to have the right and the responsibility, with all the requisite provisions and protections, to exercise their medical skill to end a life at a patient's request, just as they have maintained and improved that life up to this point.

I would do the same again, for anyone I loved who wanted to die with dignity. My deed was morally right, performed with love and trust. Why must it be illegal, fraught with anxiety and secrecy? Why shouldn't doctors assist with their care and specialist knowledge, necessary in this final act of mercy just as throughout our lives? Many, many people help their loved ones to die without the indignity or agony of waiting helplessly for the end. They must all fear criminal prosecution – and failure. It is time to review these cruel and unnecessary laws if we are serious about a humane society.

Mollie Collins

Claiming the Right to Die

I've had this insidious disease of multiple sclerosis (MS) now for twenty-six years. While the disease will sometimes progress rapidly, for me, thankfully, it has meant only a slow but nonetheless steady decline. Over the years, this has led to an increasing loss of ability to do many of the things I love. To sew, potter in the garden, run ... Running, that's a laugh when I'm getting around with the aid of two walking sticks now!

I used to relish the sun. Now its warmth leaves me weak after a few minutes. What's more, I can't even roll over when lying prone. To dance – well, Glen and I were admired whenever and wherever we were seen dancing together. All that is but a memory now. Now I can only sit, watch and enjoy the music and the atmosphere. I haven't been able

Mollie Collins was born in England and came to Australia in 1951, at the age of nine. A successful equestrian competitor and instructor, Mollie trained horses, ran her own riding school and started a 'Riding for the Disabled' group. Following her marriage to Glen, she worked alongside her husband on their dairy farm until she became incapacitated by multiple sclerosis. Glen and Mollie still live on this southwest Gippsland farm, which Mollie calls 'my little corner of heaven'. Mollie is unable to write by hand now, and uses a recently acquired word processor.

65

to walk around the farm for at least eight years, and I do miss it so much.

Before marrying Glen, I'd been running my own horse and rider training establishment, but sold it in 1968 after six years, following strong advice from a specialist who had diagnosed central vision blindness in 1967. That blindness was the first time I experienced an MS attack, though I didn't know it at the time. I then turned to freelance equestrian teaching, which left me without many of the responsibilities of having my own establishment to run.

In those days I travelled widely, as far afield as Melbourne and Deniliquin, and from far east Gippsland to Alice Springs. During this time, I was able to compete very successfully using my own horses. They were such happy and contented years.

Then I married Glen in 1970, when I was 32. He owned and ran a dairy farm in the steep and very picturesque country of southwest Gippsland.

For the first three and a half years it was an idyllic life, working alongside my husband in what I still call 'my little corner of heaven'. It was so blissfully peaceful after the hectic life I'd been living for those ten years before meeting Glen that it was quite puzzling when some strange, vague things started happening to me. I got pins and needles in my hands, and yet they felt almost numb at times. During the milking I'd feel shaky and/or weak. My right leg in particular would feel heavy, as if a weight had been attached to the boot. Strangest of all for me was the fact that I couldn't sustain the same degree of effort that had been my norm. I had been extremely fit for many years.

All these, and other things, were so intangible that some people were beginning to suspect that I was becoming a hypochondriac. After several visits to my local GP seeking answers, he told me: 'Go home, think a little more of your life on the farm with Glen and a little less of what *you* think you may have wrong with you.' Oh, that really hurt me. I have always been a positive person and never one to complain.

Cutting a very long and involved story short, it was eleven years before I was told that I had multiple sclerosis.

My first reaction was just a few tears. I quickly reassured the specialist that they were only tears of relief: at long last I knew what was wrong with me – that 'it' had a name. *Now* people might begin believing me. I'd been getting so very frustrated with my symptoms, with myself, with everybody around me.

I haven't gone through any real grieving for what was, nor have I ranted and raved and asked 'why me?' I'm of a practical nature on the whole, and it's a case of getting on with life with what you have, but I do admit to going through two or three bouts of quite deep depression in the first couple of years after being told. I did wonder how long it would be before I was reduced to relying on a wheelchair. Now, though not in a wheelchair all the time, I do need it if I have longer distances to travel. I'm very envious of amputees who have so much power in, and control of their muscles. They can do anything they put their minds to, as I would given their situation.

I have tried to stay active in as many ways as possible, although I have found I need to take rests more and more frequently as time goes on. I determined that I would *never* become bedridden: I would rather end my life than be a burden on others. That's the trouble with being too independent!

The most difficult lesson I had to learn when MS started taking over my body was to accept unsolicited help while still being gracious about it. I've never been averse to seeking help – running the riding school had taught me that – but only when I felt *I* needed it. Long ago I had decided that if ever I had a bad accident – a riding accident, a motor vehicle accident or any other accident – and was left totally dependent, unable to look after myself, then I would not want to live.

In line with this philosophy, I am at present seeking a way to end my life when the time is right. Oh, if only our laws were more humane, so that doctors could lawfully help an incurably ill person to die when life is nothing but a burden to her, and she to others!

Over the years, I have assisted my vet in ending the lives of three dearly loved animals by injection. When I saw how gently they slipped away, I determined then and there that this was the way I would wish to die. Now, because of my illness, I am even more determined than before that I shall leave this world before all the quality of my life is gone. Here I want to stress that I'm talking about quality of life *for me*, that is, about a judgment that only the sick person herself can make. It's no good if this judgment is made by others, if the person herself is able to decide. After all, whose life is it anyway?

My marriage has endured the imposition of MS, mainly, I think, because Glen and I are practical types and because we *talk* to one another. Our natures are a foil for each other – he is slow and cautious, I tend to want to have things done yesterday. We never have secrets from one another. We communicate so easily, in fact, that when I first spoke of euthanasia, although surprised, Glen wasn't too uncomfortable with the idea. Death of a loved one is not a strange experience for him. His first wife had died of breast cancer four or five years before we'd met – and we have always respected each others' deeply felt wishes.

Why is it that so many other people, including those with medical training, think that they must always keep people alive – even the very ill and infirm who earnestly desire to die? As if the wishes of the patients didn't count!

Why are we allowed to put suffering domestic pets to sleep so painlessly and without any trauma, while we ourselves must suffer the indignities of a protracted death?

It will be said that there is a huge difference between animals and people. Animals can be put to death precisely because they are merely animals. Humans are different – their lives have special worth and it would be wrong to end a human life before its time. To me this does not make sense. Humans *are* special; they are special because unlike animals they can make decisions about the way in which they want to live and die – they can *ask* for a merciful death. To deny a suffering and hopelessly ill person such a request is, if anything, *worse* than keeping a suffering animal alive.

Is it our instinctive fear of death that prevents this subject from being discussed openly? Surely our legislators and lawyers can find it in their hearts and minds to form laws that would permit the practice of voluntary euthanasia, or at least the practice of medically assisted suicide. It is absurd that our society continues to regard it as a crime if a doctor helps someone who is hopelessly racked by pain, suffering and disease to pass on into perfect peace.

While we are, in the end, but another animal species, the abolishment of an absurd law which requires humans to suffer more (not less!) than animals would be one way of putting ourselves above the animals – if this is where we belong.

I would like to end with two verses my father wrote down for me when a dear friend was dying (very painfully) of bowel cancer. I took great solace from them, as indeed did she.

ON DEATH
What's hereafter? I don't know –
Only this is certain,
This world is so beautiful
That what's behind the curtain
Cannot be any less wonderful,
And should be as exciting.

WILLING TO LISTEN – WANTING TO DIE

This cannot be the whole,
This little spot moving through space.
'Tis but a glimpse of what's to be,
When we complete the race
And enter – understanding.

J.H. Moore

My Mummy's Dying

1988. My Mummy's Dying.
The words are still with me – 'My mummy's dead. I can't get it through my head. Though it's been so many years, my mummy's dead.' John Lennon said that.

Wednesday, 16 March 1988
I leave for Adelaide in a few hours and I want to write down a few things before I go.

Mum's dying and I hate it.

Her name is Marcene Joy Theresa Ann Murphy Spears Johns.

Her maiden name was Murphy and she married my father Eric Spears when she was 19. They divorced a few years later leaving two sons – my older brother, Max, and me.

Steve J. Spears was born in Adelaide in 1951. He is one of Australia's best-known playwrights; his works include *The Elocution of Benjamin Franklin* and *Young Mo*. He has won many awards here and overseas, and also works as an actor, musician, and screenwriter for film and television.

My name is Stephen John Peter Spears. I'm a writer and probably best known for my play *The Elocution of Benjamin Franklin* but I swear to you I would rather jump off my balcony than write this piece.

A few days ago I wrote two sets of letters. One to

the *West Australian* and one to each of the State Premiers and, of course, one to Bob Hawke.

I wonder what the politicians will say? I wonder what the people will say when they read the letter?

I am so angry.

I'm not angry at death – that can be a good friend and we're all for the big High Jump sooner or later.

Not at doctors and nurses – some of them are fuckwits but most of them do a good job.

I can't be angry at Mum – she's in pain.

Why am I so angry?

THE LETTER TO THE POLITICIANS

Dear Sir,

My mother is dying of cancer and she has told me that she wishes to die before the cancer reaches her brain and while she's still sane and (thank God) in a minimum of pain.

I trust she'll be with us for a few years yet, but the odds aren't good.

As far as I understand the law in your State, if my mother decides that she's had enough, she is not legally able to ask her doctor to help her to die with dignity, (probably by a lethal dose of narcotics) as she thinks that both she and her doctor might be sued or prosecuted. Is this correct?

What is the law in your State? What are your personal feelings on euthanasia? What is your party's platform? Do you intend to change the laws or do you think they're adequate?

I understand how busy you are but **please** *regard this letter as urgent. My mother and I send you,*

Our very best wishes,

Steve J. Spears

MY MUMMY'S DYING

THE LETTER TO THE EDITOR

Dear Sir,

My mother is dying of cancer. She has told me that she wishes to die before the cancer reaches her brain and while she's still sane and (thank God) in a minimum of pain.

I trust she'll be with us for a few years yet, but the odds aren't good.

If my mother decides that she's had enough, she is not legally entitled to ask her doctor to help her die with dignity via a lethal dose of narcotics because her doctor might be sued or prosecuted. This is, I understand, the law.

Is the law correct?

If any of your readers are going through, or have had, a similar tragedy, please contact me.

> *'Peter' (Name withheld by request)*

I'm going to write an article about my reactions to Mum's death. I'll charge $2000.

Half will go to Mum, the rest will go to the Voluntary Euthanasia Society.

I'll do *anything* to please the people who read this article. I'll make them laugh, make them cry, be their clown, their private dancer, their brother, their father, their fool.

I'll write the best damn article I can and all I want from the readers is their money and one letter.

I want them to send $20 to the Voluntary Euthanasia Society in their State and a letter to their State Premier asking the Right Honourable Gentlemen to change their mongrel laws to a/ allow the use of heroin for terminal patients in extreme agony and b/ to adopt sane and humane voluntary euthanasia laws.

Be polite, reader, when you write to these curs. Just say something like 'change the laws, Mr Premier, change the laws

Mr Hawke, or I'll toss your mangy political carcass back in the kennel where it belongs.'

They're the real enemy – the pollies. The curs who govern us, the rich fat bloated complacent dogs who have the money and the connections to never have to suffer what 'ordinary' people have to suffer when they see someone they love in pain.

No, the pollies can give a 'nudge, nudge, wink, wink' to their doctors and relieve the agony of a death with no dignity.

Look out, you pollies. Steve J.'s coming to get you and you're not going to like it.

The final reason I want to write this article is to thank Mum. It's a farewell gift.

After all, it was *she* who worked as a barmaid to send me to school, to college, even to Law School.

She was just another deserted mother with two kids who worked hard, smiled a lot and made more friends in her life than most people would make in a millenium.

Mum helped to make me a writer and I want to write a piece that will make you cry.

Once she's dead, I'll need a bit of sympathy, of course, but I swear to you if any bastard who's not a family friend offers me sympathy without having sent that twenty bucks to the Voluntary Euthanasia Society and that letter to their Premier, I'll spit in their eye.

And no Scientologists or Jimmy Swaggarts or Bagwashes need apply to sign me up to your crap 'religion'.

And no junkie need tell me 'hey man, I need a fix.' Because, I'll tell you junkies something:

I hate you.

I hate you because my mum's in pain. She's in pain because she can't get heroin to ease her pain.

She can't get heroin because you half-romantic apocalyptic doom-heads who think you're suffering are running round the streets looking to get some dough for your next 'fix'.

So you pick on old people, don't you? You like to knock old ladies down and steal their handbags, don't you? You like to kick old men around, don't you? You want my video, don't you?

Come and get it, junkie.

You scumbuckets don't know what pain is.

Stay out of my way, junkie. Get yourself down to a doctor and get yourself off your habit right now because if I see you anywhere near my place I'll slice your nuts off.

That'll fix your fucking habit.

(Notes from my diary: 16 March.)

Saturday, 16 April
THE REPLIES TO MY LETTERS

Politicians
Premier John Cain (Vic.)

Dear Mr Spears,   *22 March 1988*
EUTHANASIA

The Premier has asked me to thank you for your recent letter and to advise you that the matters you have raised fall within the area of responsibility of the Attorney-General.

Accordingly, your letter has been forwarded to the Secretary, Attorney-General's Department for direct reply to you.

The Premier has asked me to express his regret over your mother's ill health.

Yours sincerely,
(signed) **name illegible**
for Peter Stewart,
Assistant Director, Justice Branch

Premier Peter Dowding (WA)

Dear Mr Spears,   *29 March 1988*
On behalf of the Premier, I acknowledge receipt of your letter about your mother.
The Premier will reply to you as soon as possible.
Yours sincerely,
(signed) D.G. Blight,
Director General

Premier Michael Ahern (Qld)

Dear Mr Spears,   *29 March 1988*
It was with sadness that I read your letter. I can understand your anguish and concern for your mother's life and comfort as she struggles with cancer.
You are correct in saying that in Queensland it is unlawful to accelerate a person's death regardless of the reasons. My party supports the existing law.
As a former Minister for Health, I have received several views on euthanasia which caused me to thoughtfully consider the matter. At present for many reasons, I believe life is precious and that humans should not have legal authority to extinguish it.
I believe euthanasia is a subject which requires much debate within the legal and medical spheres and the community generally before my Government would consider changing Queensland laws.
I take this opportunity to extend personal best wishes to you and your mother at this difficult time.
Yours sincerely,
(signed) M. J. Ahern,
Premier and Treasurer

Premier Nick Greiner (NSW)

Dear Mr Spears,   *30 March 1988*
I apologise for not replying sooner to your letter, but

the recent campaign has kept me from correspondence.

I am saddened to learn of your mother's illness and I understand her wish for peace and dignity.

Your understanding of the law is correct. However I would like to stress that considerable advances have been made recently in the care of patients suffering cancer, and in the management of pain in the best interests of the dignity of the patient.

Doctors are able to assess each case on its merits and the management of pain is given priority over possible side effects if that is the patient's wish.

I have taken up the matter with the Minister for Health, Peter Collins, who shares my concern and advises me that there are a number of hospitals which specialise in the sensitive and individual care of cancer patients. His staff would be happy to put you in contact with these hospitals if you wish to contact them.

You have raised an issue that is extremely important and sensitive and there are no plans before Cabinet at this early stage to change the legislation. We will certainly assess the issue in our first term. I know you will be aware of the moral debate that surrounds this question, although I realise that is no consolation for you or your mother in your present circumstances.

Please convey my best wishes to your mother,
Yours sincerely,
(signed) Nick Greiner, MP

Prime Minister Bob Hawke

Dear Mr Spears,   6 April 1988
Thank you for your correspondence of 12 March 1988 to the Prime Minister.

Mr Hawke was sorry to learn of the illness of your mother. Your queries regarding euthanasia have been referred to the Attorney-General, the Hon. Lionel Bowen

and he has asked to arrange for a reply to you on behalf
of the Government.
Yours sincerely,
(signed) Brendan Sheehan, Private Secretary

Premier Robin Gray (Tas.)

Dear Mr Spears,   7 April 1988
Thank you for your letter of 12 March ... I was
extremely sorry to learn of your mother's illness.

Whilst I appreciate the purpose of your approach, I
must advise that in Tasmania euthanasia is illegal by
virtue of the provisions of the Criminal code. Further, my
Government, whilst it has looked closely at the issue over
the past twelve months, does not propose to effect any
amendments ... at least not in the foreseeable future.

I respect and appreciate your concern for your
mother ... however, I must advise that my Government's
policies on this sensitive issue are firm and in line with
public opinion in this State.
Yours sincerely,
(signed) Robin Gray,
Premier

Premier John Bannon (SA)

Dear Steve,   7 April 1988
I refer to your letter dated March 12 in which you seek
information about euthanasia.

In South Australia, euthanasia is illegal. However, the
question of giving people the opportunity to determine for
themselves whether their lives should be supported by artificial support systems in the event of suffering from terminal illness has been addressed. It was the subject of a Select
Committee Report of the Legislative Council in 1980 and a
great deal of debate during the subsequent passage of the
Natural Death Act 1983 through Parliament.

The Natural Death Act 1983 enables an adult person to give directions, by signing a notice, that he or she does not wish to be subject to extraordinary measures in the event of suffering terminal illness. 'Extraordinary measures' means medical or surgical measures that prolong life, or are intended to prolong life, by supporting or maintaining the operation of bodily functions that are temporarily or permanently incapable of independent operation. The Act expressly does not authorise an act which causes or accelerates death. In other words, it does not condone euthanasia.

Since the act was brought into operation on 30 September 1984, several thousand notices have been completed by South Australians.

The Government proposes no changes to the present legislation at this time.

On a personal note I am certainly sorry to hear of your mother's illness – please convey my concern.

Yours sincerely,
(signed) J.C. Bannon

I'm still after you tax-tit-suckers and you're *still* not going to like it.

People

I got a lot of replies to my letter in the *West Australian* and to all the people who wrote to 'Peter', I thank you and Mum thanks you.

I'll only quote one of them in full.

Dear Peter,
I am a 16-year-old girl who has been through a very similar experience to you. My father had cancer two years ago. It took doctors about three to four months to diagnose this. I think if they had found out earlier it could

have been stopped. Anyway my dad died about nine weeks after having found out this tragic news. I think it was a real relief for everyone especially for my mum. My dad like your mum wished to end it all because of all the pain and suffering it was causing not only to him but to our family. At first when he was not sick I used to call him a quitter and a no hoper, trying to bring him back to life again and it worked, but as he got sicker his pain was also shared by me. I sometimes wished him dead to stop all the pain he was experiencing.

Well my dad is at rest now and I really miss him so much but he had cancer, there was nothing I could do about it and now he is out of pain and resting in Peace.

I hope your mum has plenty of strength. You must give it to her, because if she thinks strongly she will stay strong and she will live another fifty years.

Yours faithfully ...

Thursday, 12 May 1988
Mum

'I approve of Voluntary Euthanasia because I can't stand seeing people in pain. Especially *me*.

'I don't have anything against them (politicians). They want the power, they get in, then they do silly things.

'I wish people would just live their lives and be happy but so many aren't. Most people do their best. Perhaps if we cared more about *others* and less about possessions, we'd all be better off. So many people are unhappy and they shouldn't be.

'There really should be more communication between people, especially between their partners, husbands and wives and girlfriends and boyfriends, you know?

'Really, there should be more love in the world.'

MY MUMMY'S DYING

Me
The day my mother dies.
(The *Adelaide Advertiser* Death Notices.)

> **Marcene Joy Johns.**
> I'll miss you baby. Ciaou.
> Your son, Steve.

My Mummy's Dead. June 1993.

Mum died in Nov 1988. After a roller coaster of massive and increasing pain/palliative care/pain/palliative care, she died quietly in her long coma. I put the notice: 'I'll miss you baby. Ciaou' in the *Advertiser*, went to her cremation, left Adelaide on the same day and didn't go back for five years.

Mum's death boiled down to two people – Mum and me, first to Mum and her 'good death', then finally and absolutely, to me. She never asked for the promised euthanasia again, the cancer never spread to her brain and she spent most of her last months in and out of Morphineland – the Most Tragic Kingdom of Them All.

Five years.

When this book was being planned, I thought I'd write a brand new article, leap into the fray with new anger. But why? The old anger's just fine, thank you. The fray's the same. For a brief moment back then, I truly thought I could change the laws by willpower and anger alone. I was wrong.

All the old pollie players are gone – Bannon, Greiner, Hawke, Cain and so on. Now a bunch of new clowns regulate our lives and deaths. Other people have gone through similar or worse times than Mum and me. Day after day, year after year, until sane and humane voluntary euthanasia laws are enacted, the tragedies will play out again and again.

Someday, maybe, it will be my turn – or my children's.

WILLING TO LISTEN – WANTING TO DIE

Someday it will be my turn to answer the question – 'What did you do in the euthanasia wars, Daddy?'

POSTCRIPT

I wrote to the new Premier of NSW a few weeks ago.

John Fahey   *27 May 1993*
Premier NSW
Parliament House
Dear Sir,

Five years ago, my mother died of cancer. She had told me she wished to die if the cancer reached her brain, while she was still sane and in a minimum of pain.

As far as I understand the law in your State, my mother was not legally able to ask her doctor to help her to die with dignity, (probably by a lethal dose of narcotics) as both she and the doctor could have been sued or prosecuted. Is this correct?

What is the law in your State? What are your personal feelings on euthanasia? What is your party's platform? Do you intend to change the laws or do you think they're adequate?

I understand how busy you are but please regard this letter as urgent.

My very best wishes,
Steve J. Spears

Dear Mr Spears,
The Premier has asked me to respond to your recent letter concerning the Government's position with regard to euthanasia. Euthanasia is currently illegal in this State and the Government has, at this stage, no plans to change this situation.

The letter went on but I threw it away.

Janine Hosking

Death by Choice

Corny and Macca had been the best of mates since primary school. When Corny became a quadriplegic, Macca knew what he had to do. But did he take his own life as well because the law regards mercy killing as murder?

Janine Hosking is an independent documentary producer and freelance journalist. Her documentary, 'My Mummy's Dying', based on a *Good Weekend* article by playwright Steve J. Spears, was on the right-to-die issue.

A cup of warm milk just after midnight did nothing to quell Cornelis Hus's uneasiness. Two and a half hours later, after a night of broken sleep, he was jolted awake by an explosion. The realisation of what had finally happened 'hit me like a wall,' he now recalls.

In the half-minute it took for him to jump out of bed and hastily pull on pants and slippers, there was a second blast. Hus didn't hear it – all he heard was a loud thump. He remembers running the ten paces from the bedroom to the closed lounge room door. He opened it slightly. The light in the room seemed astonishingly bright.

'My son was bleeding like hell from the head. There was blood all over the sheets. I looked over to the couch where his best mate had been sleeping beside him. I couldn't see him at first, but when I kicked open the door he was lying flat down on the carpet, blood spurting from his ears. I remember saying aloud, 'Jesus, boys, why couldn't you have waited?'

In a strange, jumbled panic, Hus reached for his camera. He took time and care to line up the shots, to focus the lens. He took pictures on automatic, close-up and wide. He faltered only once, grasping his son's bed to steel himself from shaking. He knew that when the police arrived, the bodies would no longer be private property. The pictures taken, he rang the police and waited.

'The place was flooded with cops. They kept talking about a murder-suicide. I kept telling that my son wanted to die.' The irritated voice of the 57-year-old Dutchman booms through the quiet kitchen. 'I kept saying that it wasn't murder.' Even now, he still cannot believe that the police couldn't understand the difference. 'I didn't think for one moment that Macca would shoot himself as well. I think I mentioned the word euthanasia ... '

A few hours later the police allowed Hus to touch his son, the son who was named after him, and known as Corny. There was too much blood on the 23-year-old's face for an intimate goodbye. Hus kissed his son's chest. In death, his quadriplegic son's body felt cold and still – as it had in life.

Weeks later, Hus filed the slides he had taken that night and labelled the box 'Sad Case, Happy Ending ... 2.30 a.m., July 21, 1985'.

The locals have a nickname for the home of Cornelis and Maria Hus – 'Fort Hus'. It's easy to see why. Tucked away at the end of a quiet street in Winchelsea, half an hour's drive from Geelong, in Victoria, the house is all but hidden behind a high brick fence. You can't see in and they can't see out. That's the way young Corny Hus wanted it.

Smooth grey concrete, so clean it looks scrubbed, flows like an even sheet around the house, undulating at intervals over specially constructed ramps. A handrail out the back leads to a bungalow Hus built for Corny. It overlooks a neatly mown lawn, edged with perfect lines of dahlias. The only discrepancy in the nursing-home image is the chooks pecking away in the far corner of the yard.

The concrete ramps were built for Corny's electric wheelchair, the chair he never wanted to use. The bungalow was built so that he could have privacy, his very own place. Corny never looked out the kitchen window to watch his father building it. Even then, eleven months before he died, he knew he would never get to use it.

Amid all this perfection, imperfect Corny, paralysed from the neck down, had no will to live.

Hus explains why he built the fence: 'There is a swimming pool across the road, and when Cornelis first came out of hospital it was summer and the pool was being used for lots of competitions. Cornelis said he didn't want to sit on the front lawn because everyone would be looking at him. He said he was a freak. So I built the high fence and even tinted the windows of his bungalow, so no one could see him.'

Maria Hus agrees that her son was paranoid about being stared at. 'He never went out of the house except for visits to the hospital. When we put the wheelchair in the back of the car, he would make me cover it with a blanket. He would rather have my husband pick him up and carry him into the hospital than get into that wheelchair.'

The media tagged the deaths of Cornelis Hus and Wayne 'Macca' MacDonald a 'bizarre murder-suicide pact'. The Nine Network's Willesee program was so captivated by the story that it paid for both funerals, in return for exclusive interviews with the Hus family.

This was one of few euthanasia cases involving close friends. Normally this 'act of love' is carried out by a family member.

According to local folklore, Macca and Corny had become 'blood brothers' before they reached their teens. Undeniably, the 'pact' had a romantic *Boys' Own* ring to it. Wayne's older brother, Martin, recalls, 'They had vowed to grow old together, to look after each other through life, and if things went bad they wanted to go out in a big way.'

But the real story is one of a young quadriplegic let down by the system and so desperate to die that he was selfish enough to take his best friend with him. The real tragedy is the story of Wayne MacDonald, who made a naive boyhood promise, and who couldn't live with himself if he didn't carry it out.

Maria Hus and Wayne's mother, Brenda MacDonald, keep in regular contact by phone. Both are determined to fight for the implementation of voluntary euthanasia laws, and both say there is no bitterness between the families.

'I don't blame Corny for talking Wayne into the shooting,' says Brenda MacDonald. 'In this world God gives you choices. You can choose to live a good life or a bad life. Corny may have been putting pressure on Wayne, but the choice came down to Wayne. He made the decision to pull the trigger twice. We just have to accept his choice.'

Ironically, Cornelis and Maria Hus emigrated in 1955 from a country with, arguably, the world's most enlightened euthanasia laws. In the Netherlands as in Australia, voluntary euthanasia and assisted suicide are illegal. Punishment still carries a maximum sentence of twelve years, but in 1985, Dutch law was amended to allow euthanasia in cases where patients in acute distress make a well-considered request to doctors to be assisted to die. Team discussion is a prerequisite for avoiding prosecution. Those who practise it openly, at the patient's request, and in consultation with nurses and priests, are not prosecuted. Between 5000 and 6000 euthanasia cases occur annually there.

'I try to go back to Holland every three years,' said Maria

Hus. 'We seriously thought about taking Cornelis with us, so that he would be allowed to die, but my husband wanted to wait to make sure that is what he really wanted. We are accepting, down-to-earth people. I think that is why we understand so clearly why euthanasia laws are needed.'

Corny had first met Macca at the corner milkbar, a regular hang-out for the local Geelong kids. Both were still in primary school. Later, they drifted in and out of jobs and had long spells on the dole. Neither had much direction in life.

But when Corny turned 21 – by then he had a live-in girlfriend and a baby daughter – he decided he wanted to become a truck driver. Macca didn't know what his dream was.

'Macca more or less followed Corny,' said Maria Hus. 'My son had a lot of power over Macca. Cornelis did it and Macca followed.'

In July 1984, Corny got a job as a truck driver. He had saved up to gain his truck driver's licence and finally thought he had got the hang of being adult. Four days later his world was shattered when he lost control of his motorbike and was hurled into a roadside pole.

'If it had been a few inches the other way, he would have landed on the grass,' his mother explains. 'He told me he could remember lying on the ground and feeling all sensation leaving his body.' The accident broke his neck and severed his spinal cord. In hospital, a year before his death, he said to Maria, 'Remember, Mum, I died at 22, not 23.'

Although he was left with slight muscle sensation in his arms, he was totally paralysed from the neck down. The doctors hoped he might regain movement in a thumb and index finger. Says his father: 'All he wanted was movement back in his hands – he didn't want to be just a head in a wheelchair.'

An active, 22-year-old mind was hostage to a demanding

appendage - his useless body. That appendage had to be spoonfed. It urinated through a catheter, and had to have its bowels cleared manually every few days. 'The Austin Hospital [in Melbourne] was as good as it could be, I suppose,' Maria says, doubtfully. 'But he suffered indignities. One day I went into the rehabilitation ward and there were all these young paraplegics and quadriplegics lined up in their wheelchairs for their exercises. The woman who was running the session kept calling the patients her "happy little Vegemites".'

'Cornelis didn't see it as a joke, he couldn't hack it.'

Cornelis spent ten months in hospital. His friends stopped coming to see him after the first month - all except Macca, who sometimes slept beside him overnight in the hospital. Each time Cornelis came home to Geelong he became completely distraught. His parents now believed he suffered a nervous breakdown.

Says Brenda MacDonald: 'Wayne would spend all his dole money travelling on the train to Melbourne to see Corny. He would come home crying and say "Why couldn't it have been me? Corny had a job. Corny had a girlfriend, Corny had a baby ... Corny had everything."'

Cornelis's parents tried to get around the hospital system by asking the doctors to give their son a lethal injection. 'We were told that it was impossible, that it was illegal. We kept saying that it was what Cornelis wanted, he didn't want to live like that ... ' Maria stops talking, suddenly aware that her words could be misconstrued. 'Don't get me wrong, I wanted my son to live ... I loved my son ... but to make him carry on when the will isn't there is selfish.'

Attempts were made to make Cornelis's life as much as possible like the one he had lost. 'My son liked to smoke dope. I don't know about drugs, but considering his condition, I thought there was no harm in it if it made him happy. He was on so much Serapax and Valium anyway - what is the difference? My youngest son got a small amount of hash for him to eat and I hid it in the hospital. The nurses found it and called the police ... why? The police told him that if he hadn't been in a wheelchair they would have arrested him. Cornelis just laughed and said, "Take me, you're doing me a favour."'

According to his father, Cornelis didn't care who killed him, as long as it was done. By the time he left hospital and came to live with his parents, he had pleaded with everyone he knew to help him to die. 'He asked his brother, his mother, me and, of course, he asked Wayne and even Wayne's brother. I said I wanted to wait until we had finished building the bungalow. If he still wanted to die then, well, we would have to help him. But I also had his mother and the rest of the family to think about. I just wanted to wait.'

Corny clung to the hope that he would get enough movement back in his fingers to pull the trigger himself. When his girlfriend came to visit, he would make her get out his collection of rifles and polish them. In particular, they tried hand exercises to see if he could operate the trigger of his favourite gun, an antique .303 rifle. But the movement never returned to his fingers. His desperation to get someone else to do the deed became more intense.

'You know,' says Maria, 'he was constantly singing a little tune to himself in the melody of Olivia Newton-John's song, "The Banks of the Ohio". He would sing, "My .303 will set me free", over and over again.'

He even tried starving himself to death. The once strapping 1.9 metre-tall man became a pale skeleton, covered with red, weeping, pressure sores.

Macca, overcome with guilt, was finding it harder and harder to maintain control over his depression on his visits to Corny. Brenda MacDonald blames herself for pushing Macca too hard: 'I used to be constantly at him to see Corny. I kept telling him that if he didn't go nobody would. He told me that he just couldn't take it any more. I don't know when

Wayne promised Corny he would kill him. I think it was quite soon after the accident. He wouldn't talk about what he was going through – he just said he had a lot of problems.'

Soon after Macca returned to Geelong after a few months fruit-picking up north, Maria Hus decided to take a four-day break from looking after Corny. Her husband was keen to offer Macca a fulltime job as Corny's nurse and companion; Maria's holiday seemed the perfect time to test his commitment. Macca dreaded it. A few days before Maria went away, the MacDonalds' cat broke its hip. The family carried out the vet's advice and had the cat put down. 'Wayne said we treated animals better than we treat humans,' says Brenda.

During the last week of his life, Macca asked a lot of questions about euthanasia. Brenda recalls: 'We live near a school crossing which at the time was being manned by a Canadian schoolteacher. She told us that Wayne asked her what euthanasia meant. She told him all about it and then said it was against the law. At the time she thought it was out of character for Wayne to ask such an intellectual question. Just before he went to Corny's place, Wayne said that I wouldn't have to worry about him any more. I asked him if he was leaving home or if he was in trouble with the police. He just said he couldn't tell me, but that I didn't have to worry.'

Earlier, he had told a friend that he was going to kill Cornelis and himself. The friend had heard him talk about it before and didn't take any notice.

The night before the shooting, Corny and Macca enjoyed the party to end all parties. According to Corny's father, the pair drank booze and smoked marijuana until five in the morning. 'I felt uneasy about the party the whole time, but I let them go because I thought it may be the last time. I thought if they were going to do anything it would be that night.' But when Hus awoke next morning, the two were still sleeping. 'I suddenly felt better about the whole thing, I thought that maybe Cornelis was willing to live in the bungalow with Wayne and give it a go.'

The next day the district nurse was coming to show Wayne how to care for Corny. It was Wayne's day of reckoning, when he could no longer deny what his friend was going through.

'Previously, every time the nurse came, Wayne would disappear,' recalls Hus. 'That morning I made him promise that he would sit through every minute of the procedure. Before that, Wayne had never seen just how far Corny's body had deteriorated, he hadn't seen the pressure sores or watched the bowels being cleared. I think he sat through all that and then made up his mind to do what Cornelis wanted.'

That night, Hus discussed with Wayne how much money he would be paid to nurse Corny, and Wayne agreed to help him finish the bungalow. Hus told Wayne that, together, they might be able to convince Cornelis that life was worth living, or at least to give it a go for a little bit longer.

'After I finished explaining this to Wayne, he looked away and said, "But Mr Hus, Corny still wants to die."' In his mind, Macca had run out of excuses.

Neither Corny nor Macca left messages to their families. Brenda MacDonald, who still searches her son's room for clues, has found nothing.

In the early hours of Sunday morning, the death pact was carefully planned without the aid of alcohol or dope. Corny's antique .303 was loaded with the only bullet he had for it. Wayne chose a sawn-off .22 rifle with which to kill himself. Nothing was said to Corny's father, although he remembers now that Macca appeared to be agitated during the day. 'Even if I had known what was going on that night, I would have let them go. I would have told them to think it over, but they would only have been telling me what I knew anyway.'

So Macca took aim and shot his best friend. It was a clean shot. The bullet went straight into Corny's forehead. No one knows whether Wayne then killed himself because he thought his own life wasn't worth living, or because he was scared of the legal implications of what he had done. But Corny knew that Wayne was dying with him: both guns had been loaded together. In the time it took Hus to take ten steps from the bedroom to the lounge room, Wayne had picked up the .22 rifle and fired into his own temple.

Four years later, Cornelis Hus proudly shows me photographs of Wayne and Corny together. They look like a couple of larrikins, wearing shorts and singlets, carrying stubbies and guns. An old ute is nearby. But among these photographs are the slides Hus took on 21 July 1985 – horrific close-ups of bullet-shattered faces. Corny's death may have been eutha-nasia, but it was without dignity. Hus says he hasn't looked at these slides for a long time. Maria, who has looked at the photos just once, says her husband took them to show her how her son and his best friend died, so that she could see for herself the scene that continues to haunt him. One slide shows the son of Brenda and John MacDonald, splayed on the carpet, a gun by his side. Hus says he can never make up to the MacDonalds for the loss of their son: 'I see Macca as a hero – he sacrificed his life for Cornelis. He did Cornelis a great service.'

Brenda MacDonald has learnt a lot about euthanasia since the deaths. After their sons died, the families received hundreds of letters of sympathy, all of them in favour of euthanasia. Unlike Hus, Brenda doesn't see her son as a hero.

'After he died, we got a lot of people coming up to us and telling us about all the caring things he had done for them, just little things that he hadn't told us about. He was a thoughtful, sensitive boy who always went out of his way for other people, but he was just an ordinary boy, he wasn't a saint. He got into trouble like anyone else. He made the choice and did what he thought he had to do. I guess he did what anyone would do for a friend tormented with pain and misery.

'Now I want it to be legal for people like Corny to die with dignity. My son would still be alive today if Corny had had that right. I am proud of my son ... it is hard to think of what he did as a murder-suicide. I am proud of him, but he wasn't a hero.'

PART TWO

Willing to Listen

'To have denied that man help would have been an unforgivable act of cowardice and inhumanity – an immoral act.'

Sue Harper

Terminal Care in Nursing Homes

Owing to changes in our life style many more of us now die in nursing homes, often through necessity rather than choice. How people die has become one of the most complex and hotly debated issues of this century.

My own interest in the subject was stimulated, many years ago, by my encounter with two distressed old and frail residents in a nursing home who pleaded piteously with me to give them something 'to make them die', and another with a recently bereaved relative who soundly berated me for having kept her husband alive when he had wished to die. I was so moved by the evident distress of the people in both these incidents that I have spent the last twenty years, most of them as the Director of Nursing, in caring for the aged, studying end-of-life situations,

Sue Harper was born in 1915 at Colyton, New Zealand. She decided to become a nurse without ever having been inside a hospital, training at the New Plymouth Hospital. During the war she married and had three children. After her husband died she came to Australia in 1970 to be with her eldest daughter and her young family.
She returned to nursing in 1972 and was so concerned about patients who asked to die that for the next twenty years she nursed in aged care facilities, mostly as Director of Nursing in a nursing home.

and often stating and defending the case of those who want to die.

In nursing homes, as staff strive to fulfil the needs of the old and frail residents at the end of their lives, there are times when the carers find themselves in conflict with long-established concepts of care that have become outmoded by the changed clinical situation that confronts them. Nursing care itself has become a complication in the lives of those who have lived out their span and are now ready to die. It has proved to be a most effective life support system as it negates those natural causes from which people most often used to die when in their own homes – namely dehydration, hypothermia, neglect, starvation and pneumonia. (Pneumonia, of course, was once described as the 'old people's friend'.) In other words, nursing care itself prolongs the lives of residents who wish to die. Unwittingly, and with the best of intentions, we have created for some what can only be described as a horror stretch at the end of their lives.

The concern of old people generally – those not afflicted by cruel invasive conditions – is not *that* they will die, but *how* they will die. Many of them fear that they might be kept alive under circumstances where their quality of life is diminished to a level at which they no longer wish to live. For many people physical pain is not the main reason for wishing to die. There are a number of incurable conditions with a diversity of symptoms that are as much feared as pain. These are loss of independence and reliance on others, loss of awareness, loss of capabilities, loss of control over bodily functions and, most importantly, loss of control over one's life.

How universal these feelings are was confirmed by the results of a nationwide study on voluntary euthanasia and other end-of-life decisions in the Netherlands in the early nineties at the Dutch government's request.[1] This study revealed that the most common reasons for requesting euthanasia or assisted suicide were loss of dignity (57 per cent of cases), unworthy dying (46 per cent), being dependent on others (33 per cent), and tiredness of life (23 per cent). In only 10 of the 187 cases examined was pain the only reason.[2]

When I took up my duties in the nursing home about twenty years ago, the publication of Kübler-Ross's book, *On Death and Dying*[3] had kindled worldwide interest in decline and death, subjects that had been taboo until then. Lay people were beginning to challenge the paternalistic concept of care and to consider for themselves the circumstances of their own death. Voluntary euthanasia was beginning to be publicly debated. The initial reaction to it was hostile and some even thought that it was a macabre way to die.

During my years in the nursing home, not many of the residents stated explicitly and repeatedly, and in a forthright manner, that they wished to die. Among those who did voice their protests at being kept alive, the manner of expressing their feelings varied widely, as can be seen from the cases I shall describe. Regardless of how it was expressed, it was nonetheless clear that these (and some other) residents' wish to die was utterly sincere – and it was this that concerned the caregivers.

Jack Jensen[4] was by nature gentle. He was a kindly, jovial and fun-loving person, who had been an outdoor man all his life. He had become more and more frail and was now immobile with a failing heart and kidneys. He was dependent on the staff for all care.

Although he enjoyed the attention of the staff members, he saw no purpose in living as he was. 'You lovely girls spoil me,' he used to jest. 'I'm loving it, but what is the point in all of this care? This is no life for a man. My life is over now. You're keeping me going with loving kindness. Couldn't you just let me die instead? I'd be much better off.' Jack Jensen had grown tired of receiving such good care. The closing stages of his life – a man who had lived so happily until then – were tragically spent in more and more frequently repeated requests to die.

Maria Panella was of a different ilk. She was in her late seventies and mentally alert. She was quick thinking, volatile and by nature impatient. She believed in getting things done without delay and, once her dependency had reached a certain stage, she wished to die.

Maria Panella had been admitted to the home for convalescent nursing when recovering from a severe attack of pneumonia. Severely crippled by rheumatoid arthritis in her hands and knees, she had been dependent on others for all care for some time. Because of the degree of her dependency, she felt she was no longer of any use to herself or to anyone else and, for that reason, considered her life finished. (She was not the only person to express those feelings. A number of other residents had expressed very similar sentiments in nearly identical words when they had become dependent on others to what for them was an unacceptable level. Even if some of them did not explicitly ask to die, many of them did die shortly after – two, I am convinced, by a sheer act of will.)

When Maria's request to die was ignored by the staff, she decided to take matters into her own hands. 'Bring my coffin,' she would demand. 'Lower me into it and nail the lid down. It won't take long for me to suffocate. Anything would be better than being as I am.'

Outraged and indignant at her plight, this spirited woman spent the remainder of her life protesting in this manner, until she succumbed to a further attack of pneumonia.

The last days of **Alice Woods** were marked by great mental suffering at being kept alive against her will, and her concern about the cost of her care.

She had lived an active and a fulfilled life. Always frugal, Alice Woods had been careful never to waste money. Now in her early eighties, she was frail and immobile, doubly incontinent, with loss of coordination between eye and hand, and dependent on the staff for all care. In spite of her manifold disabilities, she remained an alert, practical and forthright woman.

Alice was a widow with a son and daughter, to whom she was very close. In her declining years, she had nonetheless persistently refused to live with her daughter, Helen, lest she were to hinder her career in any way. She was determined not to be a burden to her family, and it was for that reason that when she could no longer be managed from her own home she had agreed to enter a care facility.

There, for the first time she lost control over her life, a deprivation that caused her acute mental distress. In spite of the efforts of the caring staff and a concerned daughter, nothing could reconcile her to her changed circumstances.

Alice felt she had come to the home to die and she grieved constantly that her wish was thwarted. 'There's nothing I can do anymore,' she explained. 'There's nothing I want to do. Let me die.' She also objected to money being wasted on her care when she had no wish to live. 'It's a waste of resources keeping me alive. I'm finished,' she would argue. She even chided her daughter for bringing her expensive dresses and nightgowns. 'When your father was alive, I'd have been glad of them,' she told her, 'but now you are wasting money buying them.'

'Leave me alone,' she asked. 'Let me die.'

It was, however, another year before death would release Alice from her misery. It was a very long and unhappy year for her. Until the very end of her days, she continued to point out the futility of keeping her alive. It was also a long and unhappy year for her daughter, Helen. Helen was so anguished at seeing her mother so frustrated and unhappy at the end of her life, when she was powerless to help, that she sought grief counselling herself. Needless to say, the caregivers were also deeply affected by this unfortunate woman's plight.

Before admission none of these residents had been aware of

the reality of nursing home care. For many people, nursing homes remain unexplored territory. There are also those who imagine that the staff can 'let you die' or can give you something to 'make you die'. When this belief is later put into words and becomes an earnest request, the person making the request often fails to realise that she is putting a huge burden of responsibility on the caregivers, and in particular on the doctors.

Nurses are committed to delivering an accepted level of nursing care, and doctors feel that they must obey their professional ethics which requires them to preserve life. Sadly, this is often interpreted as requiring them to maintain bodily animation without regard for the person's wishes or feelings. There are, of course, doctors and nurses who strongly sympathise with a suffering patient's desire to die; but these health care professionals are unable to respond to the patient's request without fear of incurring severe civil or criminal liabilities.

The residents' terminal plight is further complicated by the fact that it is difficult for them to refuse treatment that may be prolonging their lives. In some cases, long-term, low-maintenance therapy, such as diuretics and/or cardiac medication, has been prescribed before the resident is admitted to the home. This therapy cannot be discontinued without the sometimes severely distressing symptoms and complications reccurring. Whilst these complications might eventually be lethal, people do not like to drown in their own bodily fluids, or to experience cardiac distress.

Thus some residents become stabilised at a level of bodily animation at which they can, and often do, remain for years – often senile, doubly incontinent, immobile and totally dependent. In the end, it could be said that they 'cease to exist' rather than die when their failing bodies and organs no longer respond to medication or nursing home care.

Dr Christiaan Barnard, the son of an African clergyman and

the first doctor to ever transplant a human heart, has asked: 'Have we not perverted the Christian tradition into the belief that biological existence *per se* is of supreme value and on the basis of that interpretation, sidetracked ourselves into an ethical dilemma of ghastly proportions?'[5] In the nursing home situation these words ring very true.

During those years there were two patients whose need was so urgent and their distress so acute that they were in a class of their own.

Amelia Ardman had the word 'senile' written in her case notes. There was a prevailing theory at the time that all persons over a certain age suffered some degree of senility – a supposition that would, I think, be strongly challenged today. Because of that belief, the word 'senile' was sometimes recorded on a chart before the doctor had even sighted the newly admitted resident he or she had been called to examine. While Amelia Ardman was described as 'senile', I believe she was mentally competent during those years when she so pitifully pleaded to be allowed to die. In my view, she could not have been more aware of her terminal plight, in spite of what had been written on her chart concerning her mental state.

She was in her seventies, blind and partially deaf, with a degenerative heart condition. She was also incontinent and totally dependent. Traces of her faded beauty remained on her sad and gentle face, but it was her vulnerability and helplessness that struck one so forcibly.

Her son, an educated and intelligent man, but now sad and resigned, told me that his mother had devoted the latter part of her life to the care of others. 'She who has helped so many will not now herself be helped,' he said. 'In spite of every effort to comfort and support her, she refuses to become reconciled to her disabilities. She wishes only for death. For that reason, I would support this ... this euthanasia, I believe they call it. To die is so strongly her desire. In the circumstances, it is the only humane thing to do.'

Nevertheless he understood our position, and he left saying that all he could do was to leave her in our care. I assured him we would do all we could for her – but, of course, what we could lawfully do for her was not what Amelia desired.

Amelia established that she was independent of spirit. She refused to allow us to adjust her hearing aid in the hope of improving communication with her. 'I don't want that thing in my ear,' she protested. 'Take it away. Don't torture me any further. Leave me alone.' Throughout, her dominant wish remained to die. 'Don't care for me,' she pleaded. 'Let me die.'

How often those words sounded through the ward.

At other times she would say, 'You are good and kind, but if you cared for me as you say you do, you would do as I ask. You would give me something to let me die.'

One day Dr Simmons came into the ward and was listening to this oft-repeated conversation. 'You hear what the patient is saying, Sister?,' he asked. 'She says you are good, but you're not, are you? You are the culprit, you are keeping her alive when she doesn't want to live. Is that being good? Do as she asks. Neglect her. Perhaps she will become dehydrated, develop bedsores or even pneumonia. Then she will die. It's your good nursing that causes longevity in these frail residents. Think how much more quickly people died at home without it. It appears that this patient could do without it as well.'

Dr Simmons spoke in a jocular manner, but he meant what he said. 'Yes, I suppose I could neglect her and then she would die, possibly in pain and distress.' I replied in answer to his parry. 'But what a way for a person to go in a nursing home! Nurses must nurse, and the residents should die a good death. Death from neglect is not an acceptable alternative. Don't you think this person's sincere wish to die is something for you to consider?'

Immediately Dr Simmons dropped his bantering tone and

distanced himself from the problem. 'An antidepressant is in order, and perhaps a tranquilliser,' was his only response.

I gave Amelia her first dose of the newly prescribed medication. Its rather unpleasant taste was new to her. She savoured it slowly on her tongue. 'Is this the medicine that will kill me?' she asked. 'Thank you dear. Thank you, thank you.' There was such an expression of joy on her face and such hope in her voice that I felt I was betraying her by administering that comparatively harmless potion, regulated to be given 'as necessary'.

During the ensuing years her wish to die remained constant, although the voice with its anguished plea grew increasingly faint as she became weaker. 'Let me die. Please let me die. What ... have I ... done? What have ... I ... done? Please let me die.' Day after day, week after week and month after month it could be heard. Her wish was finally granted when she died of pneumonia.

'Nature took its course,' remarked Dr Simmons righteously as he signed the death certificate.

But had it? For all those years, we had prolonged Amelia's life, against her wishes. Finally, Dr Simmons had decided not to treat her pneumonia with antibiotics, thereby allowing Amelia to die. This was not 'nature' acting. It was Dr Simmons who had finally acted. He had decided that Amelia's life should no longer be sustained, that she should receive 'comfort care only' when she might have been given antibiotics to once again stave off death from pneumonia.

Amelia Ardman, a warm-hearted, generous woman had spent the last part of her life mentally distressed because we were bound by a code of ethics that did not take into account her wish to be released from a life that no longer held any value for her. It was only when a bout of pneumonia opened a door through which Dr Simmons could admit death that her wish was finally granted.

Now, years after as I write this, her pleading words still

echo in my ears and, as a caregiver, I live with the knowledge that I failed Amelia when she was most in need. She should have been able to die when *she* had wanted to die – not when a doctor, mindful of her repeated requests to die, decided that the time had come to provide 'comfort care only'.

The mental trauma of an unfulfilled wish to die was further demonstrated by the case of **Hester Chaghall**.

She was a tall, well-preserved woman in her early eighties. To the end of her days, her arresting feature remained her vivid blue eyes, which later conveyed so eloquently what she felt when she could no longer speak.

Her life history was no different from that of many other women whose husbands had been killed in World War II. Single-handed she had brought up their two young sons, Graham and Peter who, now happily married, were successful professional men. Together with their wives and families they formed a closely knit unit, with Hester Chaghall as its much loved and respected matriarch. The strength of these family ties was one of the key elements in her case.

A forward thinking, resourceful woman still enjoying good health, she carried in her handbag a white pill that her sons understood would end her life. Her doctor had given it to her to use at a time she deemed fit, so firm was her resolve never to live in a dependent state.

Then one evening, during a family dinner, disaster struck. Hester suffered a stroke.

A stroke is much feared, and with good reason. It can occur unheralded at any time, often changing a person's life for ever. The outcome depends on the stroke's severity and on how soon the victim receives treatment after its onset.

The stroke did to Hester what she dreaded most. Not only did she become completely dependent, but she also lost control over her life. The cerebral lesion was so severe that it left her without the use of her limbs, doubly incontinent, and bereft of speech, but with an alert mind trapped in her useless body. Because she had been left so severely disabled, the opportunity to take the white pill had also been lost. (The mystery pill was never identified, nor was it ever found.)

As there was no care facility in her small country town that could accommodate her, it had been necessary to admit Hester to a nursing home which was too far away for the family doctor to visit. The sons had stressed their mother's wish to die to the doctor who had taken over her care and, although a sympathetic man, he explained that what they were asking was outside the law. He took the only course open to him, which was to keep her comfortable.

From the time of her admission, it was evident how strongly Hester objected to being as she was. Although she could not speak, she expressed her protest by being noisy and uncooperative. It was necessary to administer a tranquilliser, but it was the misery in her vivid blue eyes that caused her sons the most distress. It expressed so movingly what they already knew: that she had but one wish – to die.

There followed a most stressful time for Hester and those around her. I was moved by the sight of the son, Peter, standing at his mother's bedside with tears rolling down his cheeks. At no time is it easy to see grown men moved to tears, but there was a special poignancy in this case. 'How I dread my visits here', he confessed unhappily, 'walking up that path knowing that when I reach mother I shall find her miserable. I remember her as always being so happy, in spite of all the trials she had undergone. She deserves a better way to die than this. Isn't there anything that you can do, Sister?'

There was nothing – even though Hester's wishes were so clear, and her distress so great.

The other son, Graham, was also severely affected by his mother's plight. His wife told me that it spread a gloom over the whole family. Not as emotional as Peter, Graham felt that reason should prevail in his mother's case. 'She is so changed,' he would often remark on his visits. 'I never thought that I would see the day when mother would be so downcast. No matter how tough things were, she always managed to look on the bright side. That dejected woman with those pleading eyes bears no resemblance to the mother I remember. To see her so changed distresses me more than I can say. Keeping her alive is only prolonging her unhappiness. She shouldn't die like this. In the circumstances, can't you do as she wishes and end her life?'

I was chastened by the realisation that in a home where I was Director of Nursing, what should have been a peaceful and fulfilling event in this resident's life had become a trauma for all concerned. How could there be any dignity in such a death, I asked myself?

'Death with dignity' was fast becoming a catchword which had a comforting and reassuring ring about it. But what did it mean in exact terms, in each individual case? To Hester Chaghall it meant dying at the time when control and independence had been lost for ever. This had been her long-standing belief. But her desire to die – and with it her dignity – was thwarted by our concept of 'care', a concept which places a higher value on mere biological life than on the deeply held beliefs and values of the person whose life it is.

But why should a person die in accordance with someone else's understanding of the notion of 'care', in accordance with somebody else's values and beliefs? This question is especially poignant when raised in a clinical context where the person would have died of natural causes, had she not been 'saved', against her will, by some medical intervention. Didn't each individual know what was right for her? Because death had become 'medicalised' and 'institutionalised' did that mean that it had become in any way less personal? Did it mean that a person had lost her autonomy, the one privilege that remained to her, and therefore the most important?

I believe we must question the traditional notion of 'care'. It is difficult to imagine a more distressing situation than that faced by a person who is approaching the end of her life, who is vulnerable and dependent, yet mentally alert, and who finds herself in a care facility where her most earnest entreaty to die is ignored.

While it is often said that a person who is properly cared for does not wish to die, this is quite clearly false. Even the best of treatment will sometimes do little to quell a person's desire to die.

It is quite proper to focus first on the patients themselves. But a drawn-out and undignified dying process, endured by a patient against his or her will, can also be a profoundly distressing experience for relatives and friends. The pain and shock sometimes remain with the bereaved for the rest of their lives. Knowing that their loved ones never wished to die that way, relatives and friends often feel they have failed them when their need was greatest. Realising that they, too, may one day die in similar circumstances, they understand what peace of mind it would bring to a person at the end of life if he or she were able to maintain autonomy until the last. Many of them join Right to Die societies to further this aim. Their concern is not only for themselves but for others who must die (which in the end will, of course, be all of us), and for the friends and relatives who must witness a loved one's undignified death.

To the caregivers it is disconcerting that people who have experienced the fullness of life, who have grown old and are ready to die, should endure such frustration and mental distress at the end of their lives in a care facility, where their final needs should be addressed. Thus caregivers, too, experience a sense of inadequacy and failure. This feeling is most acute when caregivers – who wish to do all they can to support and comfort the resident – are convinced that the resident's wish to die is genuine. In this case, the resident's needs can be met only by death.

It is clear that end-of-life situations which cause such frustration and mental trauma for all involved cannot be described as satisfactory. They call into question our present concept of care, for it remains the aspiration of those who tend the dying that those to whom they minister should die a 'good death'.

What a 'good death' is in exact terms is not easy to define because situations, attitudes and needs vary so widely. Broadly speaking, a 'good death' can be described as a death that meets the needs and wishes of the dying person, and realises the hopes of relatives and friends.

However perceptive the staff of nursing homes may have become in understanding the wishes and needs of those who are approaching the end of their lives, it is not within their power to change the nature of care. It would be quite inappropriate, and contrary to the patients' best interests, if nurses were to provide less than adequate care, thereby 'neglecting the patients to death'. Helping a patient to a good death is one thing; neglecting a patient to death is quite another.

Doctors are also feeling constrained. Their ethical code and the threat of civil and criminal sanctions prevents them from acting in ways in which many of them feel they *should* be acting.

To meet their responsibilities towards the old and frail in their care, health care professionals need to re-evaluate their traditional understanding of 'care'. To truly care for a person who has reached the end of her life and who earnestly wishes to die, may require nothing less of a health care professional than to help that person to die. While many professionals already understand their role in this way, they should not be forced to step outside the law. It is therefore the law of this land which must be changed to endorse medical aid in dying.

There comes a moment when individual doctors are so moved

by the plight of the terminally ill that their resolve to respond to a patient's request to die causes them to give no thought to the consequences of their action – as it concerns themselves or the code of ethics they have pledged to uphold. So certain are they that what they are doing is right, they make no attempt to conceal their actions.

One such a trailblazer was Dr Gertruida Postma, a medical practitioner.[6] In the context of this comment on nursing home residents, it is fitting to point out that it was the mental suffering of a nursing home resident that played a decisive role in active voluntary euthanasia now being deemed appropriate treatment (under specified guidelines) for the incurably ill in the Netherlands.

Dr Postma's mother had had a stroke. It had caused partial paralysis and had also affected her speech. She was deaf and completely dependent on the staff, but her mental competence had not been affected. She repeatedly indicated that she wished to die and had attempted suicide – a case in some ways resembling that of Hester Chaghall. After much soul-searching, Dr Postma finally acceded to her mother's request. She administered a lethal dose of morphine and then reported her action to the Director of Nursing who informed the police.

This resulted in a court trial. Dr Postma was found guilty, but was given a suspended sentence and placed on probation for a year. She had stated at the trial that it was her mother's mental anguish, rather than direct physical suffering, that had convinced her she was doing no wrong.

During Dr Postma's trial, the Dutch Minister of Justice received a signed open letter from a further eighteen doctors who admitted that they had, at least once, administered a lethal dose to a suffering and incurably ill patient who had asked for help in dying.

The response of the Royal Netherlands Medical Association (RNMA) is interesting. While the Association recommended in 1973 that active voluntary euthanasia remain a crime, it acknowledged that doctors can have two potentially conflicting duties. As citizens, doctors have an obligation to abide by the law of the land (which prohibits intentional killings), but in their role as doctors their primary obligation is to the patient. When it is in a patient's interest to die, these two duties are in conflict. In such a case, doctors might reasonably decide to put their duty to the patient first.

In 1981, the criminal court in Rotterdam laid down the rules for non-criminal aid in dying. Shortly afterwards, the RNMA agreed that since voluntary euthanasia was being widely practised and not clearly wrong, it would be compatible with the doctor's professional role to engage in the practice. No doctor should, however, be compelled to practise euthanasia, if this conflicted with his or her principles. Since no patient should be disadvantaged either, patients requesting euthanasia should immediately be referred to another doctor who did not have these in-principle objections.

Provided Dutch doctors abide by the rules laid down by the Rotterdam Court, they have been, since 1981, able to openly practise active voluntary euthanasia.

In January 1990, the Dutch government commissioned the above-mentioned study on euthanasia and other medical end-of-life decisions in the Netherlands.[7] Following the commission's report, legislation was introduced into parliament in 1993, to provide clear procedural guidelines for the practice. This legislation has since been passed by both Houses of Parliament.

Here in Australia, following a worldwide trend, support for active voluntary euthanasia continues to grow. Because of public interest in voluntary euthanasia, the Roy Morgan Research Centre has regularly conducted opinion polls on the issue. The following question was first put in 1962: 'If a hopelessly ill patient, in great pain with absolutely no chance of recovering, asks for a lethal dose, so as not to wake again, should a doctor be allowed to give a lethal dose or not?' In 1962, 47 per cent of those polled gave a positive reply. This had increased to 78 per cent in 1993.[8] Other surveys show considerable support within the medical and nursing professions.[9]

Such strong support from within the community must eventually persuade our law-givers to legislate in favour of medical aid in dying for the incurably ill who request it. While community support alone does not make a practice right, there is no doubt that active voluntary euthanasia can be defended on moral grounds. As long as it remains unlawful for doctors to give direct assistance to those who are pleading to die, we can only wonder how many patients will have to continue to beg for release in vain – unless, of course, they are fortunate enough to find a doctor who is willing to risk a lot by acting illegally.

NOTES

1. P. J. van der Maas, J. J. M. van Delden, L. Pijnenborg, *Euthanasia and other Medical Decisions Concerning the End of Life*, Elsevier, Amsterdam, 1992. (For a summary of the findings see P. J. van der Maas, J. J. M. van Delden, L. Pijnenborg, C. W. N. Looman, 'Euthanasia and other medical decisions concerning the end of life', *The Lancet*, vol. 338, 14 Sept. 1991, pp. 669–74.)

2. Van der Maas et al., p. 672.

3. E. Kübler-Ross, *On Death and Dying*, Macmillan, New York, 1969.

4. All names in this article are fictitious, to protect the privacy of those concerned.

5. Christiaan Barnard, *Good Life – Good Death*, Prentice Hall, Englewood Cliffs, New Jersey, 1980, p. 89.

6. The description of this case and what follows is drawn from H. Kuhse, 'Voluntary Euthanasia in the Netherlands', *Medical Journal of Australia*, vol. 147, 19 Oct. 1987, pp. 394–96.

7. Van der Maas et al., *Euthanasia and other . . .* ', pp. 669–74.

8. Morgan Poll, May 1993, Finding No. 2436.

9. See, for example, H. Kuhse and P. Singer, 'Doctors' practices and attitudes regarding voluntary euthanasia', *Medical Journal of Australia*, vol. 148, 20 June 1988, pp. 623–27; H. Kuhse and P. Singer, 'Voluntary euthanasia and the nurse: an Australian survey', *International Journal of Nursing Studies*, vol. 30, no. 4, 1993, pp. 311–22.

Roger Hunt

Palliative Care –
the Rhetoric-Reality Gap

The Australian Association for Hospice and Palliative Care defines hospice and palliative care to mean: 'a concept of care which provides coordinated medical, nursing and allied services for people who are terminally ill, delivered where possible in the environment of the person's choice, and which provides physical, psychological, emotional and spiritual support for patients, and support for patients' families and friends. The provision of hospice and palliative care services includes grief and bereavement support for the family and other carers during the life of the patient and continuing after death.'

As a medical practitioner working in the area of terminal care for a decade, I have been confronted by numerous questions about how people should be treated as they approach the

Roger Hunt graduated from Flinders University Medical School in 1980. He has been a pioneer in hospice and palliative care in South Australia, working since 1984 in this discipline. From 1990 to 1993 he was Chairman of the South Australian Association for Hospice and Palliative Care and was closely involved in the deliberations of the Parliamentary Select Committee looking at practices relating to death and dying in South Australia. He runs courses about death and dying at Flinders University, and has published papers on terminal care patterns, resource allocation, and euthanasia.

end of life. I have encountered many challenging individual cases which have helped to evolve my thinking. I want to begin by describing one case, which shares certain features with many others, and then use this case as a focus for tackling a series of questions about the interface of palliative care and euthanasia. (The names of people in this vignette have been changed.)

John was 41 years old when he came to the Royal Adelaide Hospital in December 1989 with symptoms which had developed over the previous few months: weight loss of one and a half stone, loss of appetite and nausea, abdominal pain, small, frequent, pale bowel actions and a general feeling of malaise. Investigations revealed cancer of the pancreas with metastases (secondary spread) to the liver. This type of cancer is resistant to curative treatment and has a notoriously short prognosis, usually about three to six months from diagnosis to death. John was also recently found to be HIV antibody positive – his immediate family were aware of this but John thought most friends need not know, since he was going to die from cancer of the pancreas.

John wished to have palliative care. He was seen by a palliative care nurse at the Royal Adelaide Hospital and referred to the Southern Community Hospice Programme on 8 January 1990. He wanted his pain and symptoms alleviated, support for his family and himself, advice on care options, home nursing support and consideration for in-patient hospice care at a later stage. In hospital he had been prescribed an oral dose of morphine (10 mg, 4 hourly) which quite effectively relieved his abdominal pain, but it contributed to constipation which was successfully treated with enemas. John was keen to get home and referrals to the district nursing service and AIDS support groups, as well as to the palliative care service, were organised by the hospital staff.

The district nurse and a palliative care nurse visited John

at home, which he shared with friends Betty and Ron Moore. The nurses noted that John had been 'fairly drowsy' since commencing morphine (for pain) and metoclopramide (for nausea), and that he needed to lie down much of the time because of weakness. A few days later, John, Betty and Ron visited Daw House Hospice (the in-patient hospice unit close to where they lived) and the palliative care nurse organised a follow-up home visit with me.

John had his own clean, neat quarters upstairs in the Moore's fine home. He was a quiet, private person, realistically aware of his situation, and he spoke plainly about his wishes. His appearance clearly showed the effects of a wasting and weakening process. John complained of occasional back pain around his scapula (shoulder blade), and abdominal discomfort from an enlarged liver. He also had an oral thrush infection which was being appropriately treated. I wrote a prescription for ongoing medication, and contacted John's local general practitioner who said he could make regular home visits and was pleased to have the involvement of the palliative care team.

John spent about two weeks at home before being admitted to Daw House. During this time he could not eat much, lost more weight, and became progressively weaker and the district nurses tended a reddened pressure area on his back. He developed occasional bouts of coughing which led to dry retching, and complained of feeling distressed by his overall situation. He said, 'To be frank, I want to die, I don't want to go on.' He was emotional and tearful. He had valiantly tried to maintain his independence, and had 'tied up loose ends'.

There was little we could do to improve John's appetite, strength, and general sense of well-being. Antidepressant medication was prescribed, and counselling, good nursing and tender loving care were offered, but John remained unhappy, wishing he would soon die. Given that John was chronically distressed and that he was terminally ill, I offered him the option of sedation. If he were asleep he might not have to endure the distress he experienced in his fully conscious state. It was explained to John and his primary carers that an infusion (through a needle under the skin) of morphine (to keep the physical aspect of pain under control), and midazolam (a short-acting sedative to quell his psychological distress) might ease the suffering and induce sleepiness. The stated fact that the infusion might also have the effect of shortening his life only increased John's desire for this kind of palliation. Betty and Ron thought that this option seemed right for John and felt certain that others close to him would feel the same.

At a regular team meeting I presented John's situation for discussion. My medical and nursing colleagues considered the options and, after deep contemplation, reached a consensus that it was justified to start the morphine and midazolam infusion, but that it should be stopped for four to six hours each day so that the effects of the short-acting drugs would wear off and John would have the opportunity to talk, drink, eat, use the toilet, and say whether or not he wished to continue with the infusion.

After the infusion was started (morphine 30 mg, midazolam 30 mg and metoclopramide 50 mg), John became sleepy and barely rousable. When the infusion was stopped for a trial period, John became more alert and able to communicate. He did not like these periods and asked that the infusion be restarted: 'Just bomb me out ... I just want to sleep ... I want to die.' When a nurse suggested that perhaps his body was not yet ready to die, he replied 'I think it is.' John's loved ones also expressed the wish that the infusion not be stopped. After a few days team members agreed that the infusion should be kept going without a break.

John's condition deteriorated rapidly, but he appeared to be comfortable and calm. He became unrousable, retained airway secretions which began to rattle, and his pulse weakened. John finally died in the presence of his family and friends on the eleventh day of admission, 1 February 1990. The death certificate attributed death to disseminated carcinoma of the pancreas with a contribution from the HIV infection.

I am often asked if palliative care can always ensure a comfortable death. If the source of John's distress had been solely due to physical pain, there would have been a good chance of controlling it with medication – indeed his physical pain remained effectively controlled throughout his illness. But he experienced a range of other physical symptoms for which treatments are frequently ineffective. For example, there was little that could be done to increase his weight and strength.

The dying person undergoes enormous physical and mental changes, many of which are the source of suffering. Many terminally ill patients have a multitude of concurrent symptoms. Surveys suggest that 70 to 90 per cent of patients with advanced cancer will have significant pain that requires the use of opioid drugs.* Fatigue and generalised weakness are particularly common, and in the last few days of life, dyspnoea (difficulty with breathing), delirium, nausea and vomiting often occur.[1]

Even though the hospice movement has made significant progress in the palliation of terminal suffering, studies suggest that recipients of hospice services may be only marginally better off than non-hospice patients in terms of physical symptoms. The United States National Hospice Study, a major multi-centre comparison of hospice and non-hospice patients in the 1980s, failed to show much difference in terms of symptom control, but it did show a greater level of satisfaction among clients of hospice services.[2] However, as the principles of palliative care become integrated into mainstream health care, it is more difficult for this type of study to show differences between hospice and non-hospice patients. The

*The prevalence and severity of symptoms experienced by 100 cancer patients and the extent to which treatment helped – as reported by relatives (South Australian Parliamentary Select Committee on the Law and Practice Relating to Death and Dying, Final Report, 1992).

Symptom	Experienced? % of all cases	Severe? % of those experienced	Treatment helped? % of severe cases
Weakness	87%	75%	3%
Loss of appetite	83%	69%	11%
Weight loss	80%	71%	0%
Pain	73%	77%	75%
Constipation	58%	78%	42%
Difficulty breathing	53%	60%	63%
Trouble sleeping	48%	21%	62%
Nausea/vomiting	42%	50%	43%
Cough	42%	33%	14%
Confusion	42%	38%	0%
Fluid retention	40%	63%	40%
Other	26%	77%	25%

important point here is that even with state-of-the-art palliative care many terminally ill patients will experience substantial physical suffering.

In addition to his physical symptoms, John was experiencing intractable psychological distress. The most common types of psychological problems in patients with advanced cancer are adjustment disorders, depression, anxiety and delirium.[3] Surveys indicate that 50 to 80 per cent of terminally ill patients have concerns or troubling thoughts about death, and that only a minority achieve an untroubled acceptance of death.[4] Hopelessness, futility, meaninglessness, disappointment, remorse, and a disruption of personal identity are frequently experienced. Unfortunately, little research exists to show how much these problems can be alleviated by professional care. I suspect that many of the psychological and existential problems of dying patients cannot be solved by palliative intervention.

The hospice ideal, therefore, to provide a pain-free, comfortable death with dignity is usually unobtainable and should not be promised. It is a rhetorical myth that hospice and palliative care can relieve *all* the suffering associated with the advance of diseases like cancer, AIDS, and motor neurone disease.

Unrealistically high expectations about what palliative care can achieve may cause stress among hospice workers, and may lead to a loss of credibility with clients. The rhetoric-reality mismatch, between an ideal of care and the reality of limitations, can add fuel to the process of burnout. If the limitations of palliative care and the virtual inevitability of residual suffering are not acknowledged, then palliative carers may be spurred on to try harder and harder to relieve patients' distress, only to be further disillusioned by their efforts and filled with a sense of failure. A healthy approach is suggested by Reinhold Niebuhr's serenity prayer: 'God grant me the serenity to accept the things I cannot change, courage to change the things I can, and the wisdom to know the difference.'

Palliative care and passive euthanasia are closely linked. It was not in John's interest to try to prolong his life with artificial feeding, antibiotics or resuscitation – to keep him alive 'at all costs' – and such treatments were withheld. Indeed, it would have been contrary to his rights to force such treatments onto him, and tantamount to assault. In South Australia, as in many parts of the developed world over the past decade, legislation enabling the refusal of treatment has been enacted. John had the right to refuse so-called 'extraordinary' treatments to prolong his life, under the *Natural Death Act 1983 (SA)*.

The hospice/palliative care movement helped shift the focus of terminal care, from keeping the patient alive as long as possible to concern for the patient's *quality* of life, and respect for his or her wishes or autonomy. In this sense the hospice/palliative care movement has encouraged the widespread acceptance of voluntary passive euthanasia – where 'passive euthanasia' is understood as the act of withholding or withdrawing treatment so that the patient's life is not prolonged, and the term 'voluntary' denotes that the patient wishes this course of action to be taken. Life-extending treatment is usually not indicated in terminal care; it is usually not desired by dying patients, it may prolong suffering rather than improve quality of life, it is a misuse of precious health care resources, and withholding such treatment is a part of good medical practice.

In addition to the influence of the hospice movement, other factors have contributed to the widespread practice of passive euthanasia. These factors include an increasingly educated, consumer-orientated, aged, liberal-thinking community; a generally less paternalistic attitude of doctors, and court cases challenging the life-extension of people in a chronic vegetative state.

So, what are the steps of palliative care decision-making? John's symptoms were persistent and progressive, palliative treatments offered little hope of improving his weight, strength, psychological status, or overall quality of life, he was distressed and asking that something be done about it. Numerous articles about the type of palliative sedation given to John have appeared in medical journals and the palliative care literature.[5]

The decision to opt for the infusion of sedatives was at John's insistence – he was competent and aware of his situation. Palliative care encourages patient participation in clinical decision-making because it is the individual patient who is best placed to judge what is important to his or her own quality of life; palliative care engenders respect for patient autonomy. John's nearest carers also felt his decision was appropriate for him.

All parties involved were aware the palliative sedation might shorten John's life. This was seen by John as a positive rather than a negative aspect of the treatment. When analgesics and sedatives are infused, the patient enters a kind of 'pharmacological oblivion', and appears at peace – it is usually assumed that in this state there is freedom from pain and distress. The patient cannot eat and drink, has a dampened cough reflex, develops retained airway secretions which 'rattle' and become infected, all of which hasten death. This is also true in a subjective sense; permanent unconsciousness is, in the patient's view, similar to being dead.

It was important that the hospice team reach a consensus that John's situation justified palliative sedation. The decision was deeply pondered by the palliative care team. Based on personal perspectives, each team member regarded terminal suffering in a different way and tolerated a different level of patient distress. Differing values were accorded to treatment options. Judgements varied about the likely amount of life-shortening due to the infusion, and different weights or values were given to *quality* versus *quantity* of life. Nevertheless, a common sense of compassion and respect for John's wishes, and a reasonable level of tolerance for diverse views enabled the team to reach a cooperative decision to proceed with the infusion.

The doctor is finally responsible for the prescription of medication and may feel particularly pressured by the dilemmas that arise in these situations. If the failure of palliative care to render a dying patient comfortable and content is not realistically viewed, then the doctor may feel inadequate; not up to the hospice ideal of providing a comfortable, peaceful and dignified death. Also, a doctor may see it as right to respect the autonomy of the patient, but believe that it is wrong to deliberately accelerate the process of dying or to transgress the law on taking life.

The doctor risks the possibility that someone who is only vaguely acquainted with the terminal phase – perhaps a religious-fundamentalist daughter who arrives from interstate, feeling guilty because she was not present earlier, and discovers that the patient's last breath was accompanied by substantial doses of medication – could point an accusing finger and say, 'You killed my father!' The doctor may fear being hauled before a court on charges of killing the patient.

The existence of this possibility, and the threat it poses to the doctor, may prevent some patients from receiving appropriate palliative care. An improved legislative framework is required to protect palliative carers from criminal or civil liability when a treatment has the effect of shortening the patient's life – provided the treatment is in accordance with the wishes of the patient, is given in good faith, without negligence and in accordance with appropriate standards of palliative care. Such legislation would give palliative care patients, doctors and nurses greater licence in choosing appropriate methods to treat suffering at the end of life.

The next question is fundamental and perplexing: is voluntary euthanasia morally different to palliative care?

Many hospice advocates are now willing to admit that some palliative treatments (such as the treatment John received) can hasten death but they are keen to draw a moral distinction between these kinds of treatment and active euthanasia. This distinction uses the principle of double effect and hinges on the *intention* of the treatment. According to the principle of double effect, the intention or 'primary effect' of palliative care is to relieve suffering, while any effect on the timing of death is merely secondary, unintended and incidental. By contrast, with voluntary active euthanasia, a quick death is desirable, and intended.

The principle of double effect, however, fails to make a

moral distinction between palliative care and active euthanasia for three reasons. Firstly, a most striking feature of the intentions of both palliative care and voluntary active euthanasia is that of *compassion*. Both practices are morally equivalent in that virtuous humane motives underlie the effort to ease suffering in the way desired by the victim of disease. This is clearly different to murder and manslaughter where sinister motives and recklessness prevail against the wishes and interests of the person who is killed.

Secondly, the principle of double effect tends to deny that an early death as a result of palliative treatment may actually be desired and intended by the patient and carers. If the patient and carers opt for palliative sedation, knowing that this will have the effect of shortening the patient's life, and the treatment is intentionally administered, then the claim that there was absolutely no intention to shorten the patient's life would be less than honest. Dr Timothy Quill has raised this issue of multilayered intentions and the need for honesty: 'Our current ethical thinking and legal prohibitions reinforce self-deception, secrecy, isolation, and abandonment at a time when the exact opposite is needed.'[6]

Thirdly, the accelerated death of a patient receiving palliative sedation is not merely tenuously connected or incidentally related to the treatment, as the principle of double effect suggests, but is actually *caused* by it. Death is a direct consequence of palliative sedation, as it is with the administration of a lethal injection in euthanasia, only in the former case it is slower than in the latter. Rather than being morally distinct entities, therefore, these two practices are related on the same continuum of end-of-life care, and palliative sedation can be regarded as a form of 'slow active euthanasia'.

The principle of double effect, by ignoring or diminishing the causal connection between the treatment and the hastened death, dangerously undermines the acceptance of professional responsibility for this outcome of treatment. Good clinical

practice demands that the important consequences of treatment options be considered and discussed with clients. In
terminal care, as in any other area of medicine, it is not
acceptable to focus purely on the intended outcome of
treatment while disregarding the other effects of the treatment.
It is poor clinical practice as well as morally evasive to simply
turn a 'blind eye' to the fact that a palliative treatment may
shorten life.

It seems to me that the principle of double effect is a
psychological construct or a *psychological defence mechanism*
which enables clinicians to intervene in suffering with life-
shortening acts while appearing to defend or guard the sanctity-
of-life principle. The principle of double effect serves a useful
purpose if it maintains a sense of integrity among clinicians
who cannot bear the idea of actively assisting a patient to
die, and it cannot be completely disposed of for this reason,
but it does not sustain moral arguments against active
euthanasia.

Active euthanasia flagrantly breaches the sanctity-of-life
principle. The fundamental moral issue is whether the sanctity-
of-life principle should be absolutely inviolable, or whether it
can be breached. There are many examples of breaches: self-
defence, capital punishment for retribution and as a deterrent,
termination of pregnancy, political and religious wars and so
on. There is perhaps no better justification for breaching the
sanctity-of-life principle than to fulfil the request of a dying
person who is suffering.

Therefore, do hospice patients request a quicker terminal
course? Despite our efforts, John judged his quality of life to
be overwhelmingly poor and he had a clear resolve that his
life should end quickly. His situation was unbearable to him.
Who is better placed than the person who is suffering to judge
whether or not his suffering is bearable?

Some hospice advocates believes that palliative care is
capable of negating the desire or need for voluntary active

euthanasia.[7] Some believe that requests for medical aid in dying could only reflect inadequate palliative care, a lack of love, depression, and/or cultural weakness.[8] But even with the best palliative care there may be considerable residual suffering, a point I made earlier, and requests for euthanasia continue to be made.

Rather than 'do hospice patients request euthanasia?' the question should be 'how often?'. Unfortunately, this question has not been widely researched, but data obtained at Daw House Hospice over a two-year period give some indication. In this survey, staff who attended a weekly death-audit meeting were asked to recall the spontaneously expressed views of patients. Of the 331 patients who died during the study period, 77 per cent never mentioned a desire for a quicker terminal phase, 11 per cent said 'I wish it would hurry up', 6 per cent asked a staff member 'Could you hurry it up?' and 6 per cent made a clear, persistent request for a quick death.

Some requests for a speedier death may have been missed. There was no systematic attempt to elicit patient views. The views recalled were spontaneously expressed, in a setting where deliberate euthanasia is not countenanced and not practised. It is possible that some patients who harboured a desire for a speedier end to life saw little merit in expressing this to staff. Many patients were admitted in a moribund state and were unable to state their wishes. Also, many members of the hospice team, particularly nursing staff and volunteers, were unable to be present at the audit meetings to report what may have been said to them. These factors would tend to inflate the 'never mentioned' category and cause underestimates in the other categories.

Should active euthanasia be included as a form of palliative care? In answer I will use this analogy: a person with a terminal illness is like someone dangling from a rope over the side of a cliff who cannot be hauled up; passive euthanasia is letting the person hang until he or she falls off, whereas active euthanasia is cutting the rope to expedite an end to the person's distress. In John's case the rope was cut 'slowly'. Advocates of voluntary euthanasia argue that the dangling person should have the option of having the rope cut to allow a speedy end.

When the well-being of a terminally ill person is adversely affected by continued existence, when there is no hope of improvement in a poor quality of life, and when relief is persistently requested by that person, the optimal form of palliation may be to administer a lethal medication. The best palliative care option is one which serves the interests of the patient, provides effective relief of suffering, accords ample respect for the patient's autonomy, and, ideally, has the support of those people who are close to the patient. Active voluntary euthanasia may be the most compassionate and best option in some situations. Clinical as well as moral imperatives, therefore, may at times compel a palliative care doctor to perform active voluntary euthanasia in the interests of the patient.

So, why has the hospice movement traditionally rejected active voluntary euthanasia? Partly because Christian idealists led the development of the hospice movement (they named services to honour saints), and active euthanasia conflicts with the sanctity-of-life principle as espoused by many religious groups. Dame Cicely Saunders, the 'founder' of the modern hospice movement who opened St Christopher's Hospice in 1967, for example, as a young woman 'went through a period of evangelistic fervor, during which she was a Billy Graham counsellor, before she finally settled into the Anglican church.'[9] Hospice rhetoric such as 'Hospice care neither hastens nor postpones death, but seeks to affirm life so that one can live fully until death occurs'[10] appealed to the 'right to life' lobby group which polarised itself against the concept of medically assisted death.

The early hospice movement needed to gain medical

respectability. It did this by creating an image of the ideal or preferred state, and by promoting the successes of the emerging discipline of palliative care. The evangelical fervour of the early hospice movement led to claims that nearly all the suffering of terminal illness could be controlled, and this negated any need for active euthanasia. Besides, during the hospice movement's formative years, death was regarded as something of a taboo in mainstream medical culture, and although hospice care inevitably evokes images of death, any association with the killing of patients would have seriously undermined medical respectability. The rejection of euthanasia enhanced the respectability of the hospice movement, it ensured the support of religious organisations and furthered the acceptance of hospice principles by conservative health care professionals.

As palliative care has gained respect as a discipline of medicine, and as it has become integrated into the system of health care, it has become less influenced by Christian idealists and more influenced by the secular scientists. The new leaders of the hospice/palliative care movement are specialist doctors with academic standing. Reduced religious influence, newly gained medical respectability, and increasing exposure of the limitations of palliative care by scientific methods have weakened the movement's formal rejection of voluntary euthanasia. Caution, rather than outright rejection, is the current attitude, as indicated by the comments of Dr Ian Maddocks, Australia's first professor of palliative care: 'The quick fix aspect makes me cautious ... we should defend ourselves against a "culture of fatal attraction" which would make opting for earlier death the right and noble thing to do.'[11]

Most dying cancer patients are unlike John – they do not want a quick exit – and palliative carers have greater opportunity for exchange and for offering loving support. Palliative care workers are frequently pleased at what can be achieved when their knowledge and skill is combined with persistence and compassion. They fear that if the 'quick fix' became a cultural imperative then the potential for the positive responses to palliative care would be limited.

Nonetheless, the euthanasia and hospice movements have much in common. Both have been driven by similar forces, and have continued to grow. The increase in death awareness and interest in terminal care during the latter third of the twentieth century has been fuelled by the increasing numbers of people who live out their natural life span, the aging of the population, a shift in the causes of mortality to the degenerative diseases of the aged, the improved ability of modern medicine to prolong the terminal phase of life, a disenchantment with the application of biotechnology in terminally ill patients who have a diminished quality of life, escalating health care costs, a desire for more humane care at the end of life, and a concern for the rights of the terminally ill.

Both movements aspire to effecting a 'good' death, and both have adopted the slogan 'death with dignity'. Both movements focus on the 'rights of the terminally ill', and attempt to give a voice to the concerns of many who are worried about the quality of life of the terminally ill. Both movements emphasise compassionate, humane care, and the central role of patient participation in decision-making. A full or holistic assessment of the patient's physical, emotional, and spiritual dimensions, and the wishes of close family and friends, are regarded by both as essential to establishing the appropriateness of interventions. Unlike the curative mode of care, in which the use of invasive investigations and treatments can be justified by the potential benefit in terms of life-years saved, the palliative and euthanasia modes of care give priority to quality of life – as death becomes imminent, treatment aimed solely at prolonging life is considered to be increasingly 'burdensome' or 'extraordinary', and generally not of the kind to enhance the quality of the patient's life.

Do these trends in terminal care suggest that medical aid in dying will become more openly accepted?

A gradual transition in the values of medicine has taken place; from the values of the 'curative' mode of care, which aims to extend life even during the terminal phase, to those of the 'hospice/palliative' mode. This transition has effectively diminished adherence to the practice of keeping dying patients alive at all costs. It has shifted the emphasis of care toward *quality* rather than *quantity* of life.

The euthanasia mode requires even more concern with quality of life, as judged by the patient, relative to the quantity of life. For active euthanasia to occur, the burden of concern about lingering suffering must overwhelm concern for the continued life of the patient.

The principle of autonomy was neglected in terminal care before the development of hospice and palliative care – most patients were ill-informed of their situation, and they were submissive to medical paternalism. The palliative mode emphasised the importance of sensitively informing patients about their state of health and the treaatment options available to them, and stressed the importance of patients being involved in decisions about their quality of life. The shift to the palliative mode, therefore, moved the power base in the relationship between health carers and patients, from professional domination to increased patient autonomy.

However, the traditional mode of hospice care, by denying the patient's wishes for medically assisted death, has placed a serious limitation on patient autonomy. The availability of voluntary active euthanasia would extend the autonomy of terminally ill patients.

Trends in the evolving values of terminal care, therefore, suggest that palliative care may eventually expand to embrace the practice of voluntary active euthanasia. The continued maturation of the hospice/palliative care movement, an increasing recognition of its limitations and of the extent of residual suffering, and a broadening of palliative techniques to include treatments which have the effect of hastening death, are closing the gap towards fast-stream active euthanasia.

Meanwhile, euthanasia advocates support the provision of palliative care, and they consider medically assisted death as an extension of, rather than an alternative to, good palliative care. Medically assisted death is seen as the last option, to be used only after other palliative care efforts have been tried and failed or are considered unlikely to help the patient.

The evolving social context also suggests that palliative care will include medical aid in dying. Individual responsibility for making choices is likely to increase as society becomes more liberal, less influenced by religious authority, and more oriented to the plurality of needs. Public opinion shows that an increasing majority favours the availability of this option for terminal care. The Roy Morgan Research Centre has published the responses of Australians which show that about three quarters of the population now favour medical aid in dying, as opposed to surveys of twenty years ago which showed about half the population in favour.*

Public interest in these issues naturally includes interest in the Netherlands, so far the only country in the world to openly practise voluntary euthanasia. Socially and culturally, the Netherlands is highly evolved, and there is an open attitude to hitherto forbidden topics such as death. The Dutch possess a strong sense of order, liberty, and responsibility. They are generally well-educated and sensitive to human rights issues. The health system provides egalitarian access, it is regarded by the World Health Organization (WHO) as one of the best

*Responses of Australians to a question about voluntary active euthanasia: [expressed in percentages]

If a hopelessly ill patient, in great pain with absolutely no chance of recovering, asks for a lethal dose, so as not to wake again, should a doctor be allowed to give a lethal dose, or not?

Year	1962	78	83	86	87	89	90	91	92	93
Give dose	47	67	67	66	75	71	77	73	76	78
No dose	39	22	21	21	18	20	17	20	18	15
Undecided	14	11	12	13	7	9	6	7	6	7

in the world, and it has a strong primary care component. The principles of palliative care, rather than being sequestered in free-standing hospice units, are integrated into the mainstream of health care delivery. Dutch doctors are greatly respected and trusted – during World War II they resisted Nazi efforts to coerce them into wrongful killing. There is no evidence to suggest Dutch doctors have lost respect from the community for practising active voluntary euthanasia – a profession is as great as the responsibilities it takes on, and as good as the quality with which it discharges those responsibilities.

Experience in the Netherlands suggests euthanasia practices are not undertaken easily or lightly – these practices cannot be regarded as a 'quick fix' or a 'fatal attraction'. According to a comprehensive study commissioned by the Dutch government, over 25 000 patients per year seek assurance from their doctors that they will assist them if suffering becomes unbearable.[12] Of these, there are about 9000 explicit requests for voluntary euthanasia or assisted suicide, of which less than a third are agreed to. Only about 3 per cent of all deaths in the Netherlands involve active euthanasia. In most cases palliative alternatives are found which make life bearable again, or death intervenes before any action is taken.

Most cases of euthanasia (85 per cent) involve cancer patients, and only about 8 per cent of cancer patients have euthanasia. The patients make requests because of loss of dignity (57 per cent), pain (46 per cent), being dependent on others (33 per cent), or tiredness of life (23 per cent). In only 5 per cent of cases was pain the only reason. Medical complicity remains difficult when a persistent request for euthanasia is made: 'And we always hesitate! In all cases we will after a request for euthanasia try to improve our palliative care to avoid the need for euthanasia. And in all cases we will try to understand why this patient chooses death over life ... euthanasia can only be done as the last dignified act of terminal care.'[13]

What can we conclude from this discussion? Palliative care has improved the care of the dying, but there are some patients for whom the current repertoire of palliative treatments seems inadequate. John's case shows how difficult it is to treat problems such as weight loss, weakness, and the loss of independence. John wished for a quick end to his life, but legal prohibition prevented euthanasia from being an option.

John received a sedative infusion which eased his distress and hastened his death. This type of palliative care is now widely accepted, and the principle of double effect is used to justify the shortening of life caused by this treatment. I have argued, however, that this doctrine fails to make a moral distinction between the 'slow' euthanasia of palliative sedation and the 'fast' euthanasia of a lethal injection. In some circumstances it may be more compassionate and appropriate to accede to the patient's wish for the fast form of euthanasia.

Social evolution and the maturation of the hospice movement have resulted in growing public and professional acceptance of treatments which improve quality of life at the expense of quantity of life, and of voluntary active euthanasia. In the future, people in situations similar to John's may have the reassurance of an improved range of choices for their care and greater control over the ending of their lives.

NOTES

1. G. Johanson, 'Symptom character and prevalence during cancer patients' last days of life', *American Journal of Hospice and Palliative Care*, 1991, 8; 2, pp. 6–8.

   V. Ventafridda, C. Ripamonti, F. De Conno, M. Tamburini, B. Cassileth, 'Symptom prevalence and control during cancer patients' last days of life', *Journal of Palliative Care*, 1990, 6:3, pp. 7–11.

   F. J. Brescia, D. Adler, G. Gray, M. Ryan, J. Cimico, C. Mamtani, 'Hospitalized advanced cancer patients: a profile', *Journal of Pain Symptom Management*, 1990, 5(4), pp. 391–97.

   E. Curtis, R. Krech, T. Walsh, 'Common symptoms in patients with advanced cancer', *Journal of Palliative Care*, 1991, 7(2), pp. 25–29.

   N. Coyle, J. Adelhardt, K. Foley, R. Portenoy, 'Character of terminal illness in the advanced cancer patient: pain and other symptoms during the last four weeks of life', *Journal of Pain Symptom Management*, 1990, 5, pp. 83–89.

   D. Reuben, V. Mor, J. Hiris, 'Clinical symptoms and length of survival in patients with terminal cancer', *Archives of International Medicine*, 1988, 148:7, pp. 1586–91.

   R. Fainsinger, M. Miller, E. Bruera, J. Hanson, T. Maceachern, 'Symptom control during the last week of life on a palliative care unit', *Journal of Palliative Care*, 1991, 7:1, pp. 5–11.

   P. Henteleff, 'Symptom prevalence and control during cancer patients' last days of life', *Journal of Palliative Care*, 1991, 7:2, pp. 50–51.

2. V. Mor and S. Masterson-Allen, *Hospice Care Systems: Structure, Process, Costs and Outcome*, Springer Publishing Co., New York, 1987, p. 116, pp. 125–76.

3. L. Deragitis, G. Morrow, J. Fetting et al., 'The prevalence of psychiatric disorders among cancer patients', *Journal of the American Medical Association*, 1983, 249, pp. 751–57.

J. Bukberg, D. Penman, J. Holland, 'Depression in hospitalized cancer patients', *Psychosomatic Medicine*, 1984, 46, pp. 199–212.

4. M. Vachon, B. Conway, W. Lancee, W. Adair, 'Final Report on the needs of persons living with cancer in Quebec, Toronto', Canadian Cancer Society, 1991.

    J. Hinton, 'Comparison of places and policies for terminal care', *The Lancet*, 6 Jan. 1979, pp. 29–32.

5. E. De Sousa and B. Jepson, 'Midazolam in terminal care', *The Lancet*, 1988, 2:9, pp. 67–68.

    B. Amesbury and K. Dunphy, 'The use of subcutaneous midazolam in the home care setting', *Palliative Medicine*, 1989, 3, pp. 299–301.

    P. McNamara, M. Minton and R. Twycross, 'Use of midazolam in palliative care', *Palliative Medicine*, 1991, 5, pp. 244–49.

    D. Bottomley and G. Hanks, 'Subcutaneous midazolam infusion in palliative care', *Journal of Pain Symptom Management*, 1990, 4:5, pp. 259–61.

    A. Burke, P. Diamond, J. Hulbert, J. Yeatman and E. Farr, 'Terminal restlessness – its management and the role of midazolam', *Medical Journal of Australia*, 1991, 155, pp. 485–87.

6. T. E. Quill, 'The ambiguity of clinical intentions', *New England Journal of Medicine*, 1993, 329, pp. 1039–40.

7. K. Rayner, 'Euthanasia: dilemma of a community', *Australian Family Physician*, 1993, 22:3, pp. 545–51.

8. L. De Souza, 'Euthanasia', Paper presented at the First International Hospice Conference in India, 1991.

9. D. Brand, 'Dying with dignity – profile on Cicely Saunders', *Time*, 12 Sept. 1988, pp. 90–91.

10. M. Manning, *The Hospice Alternative: Living with Dying*, Souvenir Press, London, 1984.

11. I. Maddocks, 'Euthanasia debate: Resisting the fatal attraction', *South Australian Medical Review*, 1992, (Publication No. SBG 0499, ISSN 1033–1239).

12. P. van der Maas, J. van Delden, L. Pijnenborg, C. Looman, 'Euthanasia and other medical decisions concerning the end of life', *The Lancet*, vol. 338, 14 Sept. 1991, pp. 669–74.

13. P. Admiraal, 'Euthanasia in a general hospital', in A. Smook and Vos-Schippers (eds), *Right to Self-determination*, University Press, Amsterdam, 1990, p. 106.

The Case of Miss T.

The following is an edited transcript of a discussion at a seminar on the theory and practice of ethics in medicine. I am grateful to Dr John Wiltshire for his helpful comments and suggestions. The participants included doctors, nurses, social workers, philosophers and laypeople with an interest in ethics. It is included here because it illustrates well how finely balanced the clinical relationship is and how unpredictable its course can be – even when the patient is clear about his or her wishes to die and the clinician tries hard to be open and responsive.

Paul Komesaroff is a physician and medical researcher at the Baker Medical Research Institute in Melbourne, where he is also Executive Director of the Eleanor Shaw Centre for the Study of Medicine, Society and Law.

PK: I'd like to tell you about the case of an elderly woman I once looked after and to ask your opinions about what I should have done at the time. It was a difficult and complex case, which made a big impact on me – indeed, even today, years later, scarcely a day goes by without some aspect of it recurring to me in one way or another.

I was working as a medical registrar at a large public

hospital at the time. The patient, whom I eventually came to know very well, had already been seen over many years at the hospital. She was regarded as something of a medical curiosity because she had a collection of odd conditions, thought to be autoimmune in character – that means that the body turns on itself and attacks its own tissues. When I first met her she was 78 years old. She had a long history of rheumatoid arthritis, which although it was no longer active and no longer caused her pain, had left her body ravaged and debilitated.

She had also a condition called 'Sjögren's syndrome', which causes dry eyes and mouth and commonly accompanies rheumatoid arthritis, chronic liver disease (diagnosed as so-called 'chronic active hepatitis' years before) and a chronic lung condition, also thought to be autoimmune in character, called 'fibrosing alveolitis'.

As I said, the rheumatoid arthritis had left her body badly deformed, but it was really the lung condition that caused her the most problems. It made her breathless – so much so that for years she had been unable to walk more than a few steps at a time – and it affected her heart, so that she retained fluid in her legs and her lungs.

She took a large number of medications, which for a considerable period had served her very well. In spite of her physical limitations she remained mentally active and alert, and indeed, managed to tend the garden in her small house, of which she was justifiably proud. I visited her house once – using some excuse, because I'd heard her talk so much about it and was curious. She'd lived there for nearly forty years, and it was her whole world, which she had fashioned lovingly and with great care and subtlety. The garden too was a source of joy to her, and she proudly showed me around her rose garden and her vegetable patch.

Miss T. had never married and had lived almost all her life alone. Evidently, she had been somewhat of a rebel in her day – certainly, a 'modern woman'. She had decided early that she would have an independent career, and she went to university where she gained a degree in English. She later became a teacher and eventually was a respected English Mistress at a private school for girls. Literature was her life and her love, and she could speak for hours about books she had read and places she had visited in her imagination.

Apparently she had had a number of relationships and her liberated lifestyle had in its day raised a few eyebrows. But she never compromised her independence. She bought her own house and supported herself, even in the face of her considerable medical problems.

I didn't ever find out much about her family. In fact, the only family I came to know about was an elderly sister, to whom she remained close all her life, and a niece. Her sister, who was 82, herself suffered from osteoarthritis of the hips, which, together with her considerable obesity, substantially limited her mobility. She lived a few kilometres away. The niece was in her late twenties or early thirties and, I think, was still a student. She had developed quite a close attachment to her aunt and visited her every week or so and helped with shopping and cleaning. Incidentally, I should mention that for years Miss T. had received the maximum available community supports, including council help, 'Meals on Wheels', visiting nurses when required and so on.

The story that I want to share with you started some time before I knew her. Miss T. had been going to a GP for many years – he was almost as old as she was. They had come to know each other reasonably well and would often chat about current affairs and books they were reading. As I understand it, on a number of occasions she had raised with him the possibility of her becoming so disabled that she would no longer be able to care for herself. She stated directly and unequivocally many times that if she were to lose her independence she would not want to go on living. She had said to the doctor that if she could no longer follow the style of life of her choice she would want him to give her something to help her die.

Well, it so happens that her condition gradually deteriorated, to the point where it was apparent to the GP that she could no longer reasonably manage at home on her own. Furthermore, given the inexorable nature of her condition, it was clear to him that in due course she would require quite substantial nursing support. Accordingly, he told her that he thought the time had come where she had to seriously consider entering a nursing home. Miss T. replied something like: 'We have discussed many times how my independence is most precious to me. I don't want to go on living in circumstances in which my lifestyle is not of my choosing. Please give me something to make me die.'

I'd like you to imagine that you are the local doctor. What would you do? What should he have done? Before answering this, perhaps if anyone has some factual questions they would like clarified we should do that first.

A: I have two small questions. First, what sort of medications was she taking?

PK: She was taking digoxin, frusemide (a diuretic), captopril (a medication for cardiac failure) and inhaled Ventolin as needed. I think that was all.

A: And how disabled was she was at this time? I mean, could she walk, use her hands and so on?

PK: This was a bit before I knew her, and I can really only speak about the later time in detail. But as I understand it, at that point she really couldn't walk more than a few steps at a time without getting short of breath. Her hands were distorted and she had had to have special taps put into the house and that sort of thing, but that was a chronic problem which I don't think had changed much for some years.

If you were the GP, what would you do in his position?

B: It's hard to answer without being there, but it if it's her wish to die – and it seems that she's thought it out carefully and it's not just a spur of the moment thing – then she should be able to do as she pleases. I mean, she's an autonomous person, isn't she, and she has the right to decide whether she will live and die.

C: But she's actually asking the GP to help her and that's another thing. If I was her GP I think I would find it very hard to help her, especially after knowing her all those years.

D: I don't think that she has the right to ask the doctor to kill her. Anyway, that's not his job. She's asking him to do something that has nothing to do with doctoring.

B: I disagree with that. The doctor's job is to relieve suffering, and this woman is suffering. Helping her die would just be a continuation of what he'd been trying to do all along.

E: No. The doctor's job is to preserve life, not to take it. To kill her would be to betray everything that medicine stands for. Anyway, if she really wanted to die, she could do it herself – she could just go away and take poison, or something.

F: But she might not know how to do it. A lot of people don't. Anyway, if she tried and failed, it could be very distressing.

PK: I think some of that is true. When I knew her, she would often say that her independence and her books and so on were very important to her, but that she never wanted to suffer. 'I've never liked pain', she once said to me, with her characteristic irony, 'yet I've had so much of it.'

B: D, don't you think that it should be her choice whether she lives or dies? She is a mature adult. Why shouldn't she make up her own mind?

D: It is not that she shouldn't make up her own mind; it is that she is imposing on the doctor to kill her. I think that's wrong.

G: *(With intensity)* I think it's the other way round: it's the doctor who's on the power trip. I really can't see what the point of this is . . .

F: Perhaps the doctor doesn't actually have to kill her, but could tell her what to do, how to do it quickly and painlessly ...

B: Perhaps he could give her a normal prescription of pills and tell her that if she took all of them at once it would kill her.

F: That's a bit like the suicide machine we were talking about earlier today, isn't it? It would then be her decision and she would be carrying it out.

E: I'm very surprised by the way this discussion is going! Everyone has assumed that because she has said that she wants to die once that's all there is to it ...

B: She's said it on many occasions ...

E: People say all sorts of things when they are sick or distressed. She's probably upset that he's told her that she has to go and live in a nursing home. I know I would be. It's natural for her to think about ending it all. But she might change. She might get to like it. She hasn't even tried it out.

PK: So, E, what would you do if you were in the situation of the GP?

E: Well, I'm not a doctor, but I suppose you'd have to talk with her and make her understand that it's not the end of the world, but that she's just entering a new phase of her life. It may even turn out to be very satisfying for her. In particular, it might bring her closer to God, if she's religious.

B: *(Becoming heated)* Look, I think that that's just incredibly paternalistic! She's made up her mind and we have to respect that.

PK: What would you do, B?

B: I wouldn't kill her outright because I don't want to go to jail, though if I could do it legally I would. I don't think there's any difference between giving someone pills to kill themselves and giving them an injection, except that the injection would probably work better! In the circumstances, I'd probably give her some tablets or tell her what tablet to take or something like that, like F suggested. But I think she's got the right to die if she wants to.

(Calls of 'No!' and 'You can't kill her!')

PK: Unless I'm wrong, B and F are in the minority. Although a number of you are in sympathy with her wish to die, no one else would take active steps to kill her or to facilitate her death. Is that right? Well, it so happens that the GP refused to help her die. I suppose you already guessed that: if he hadnt, there wouldn't have been a story for me to tell.

The GP refused and she went home. A few days after this she was admitted to hospital, and this was when I met Miss T. for the first time. She had an exacerbation of her lung and heart conditions. When I first saw her, she was certainly in a bad way. She had severe oedema, that is, fluid retention, extending from her feet right up to her waist. She was so short of breath that she literally could not sit up without gasping for air, and she was certainly unable to stand up or walk. All this was superimposed on her tiny, emaciated body with its characteristic distortions from chronic rheumatoid arthritis.

During her stay in hospital, which lasted about four weeks, I came to know her quite well. In spite of her debility, she was an engaging and lively woman who loved to talk about life and people. She gave me an account of her earlier life – her determination to live the way she wanted and not to conform to the stereotypes of the times, not to marry or become a housewife. She was proud of her achievements too. As I said before, she loved her home and her books, and was never happier than when talking about some work of literature that an event or circumstance had reminded her of or quoting an apt verse of poetry. She painted a vivid picture of her own life, and of what had driven her. 'I've drunk life to the lees,' she used to say somewhat grandiosely. 'I've been happy and I've suffered too.'

I think I'm not being too immodest to say that Miss T. came

to regard me as a kind of surrogate grandson – and the warmth was mutual.

D: Did she ever discuss with you her wish to die?

PK: No. She never raised that question directly, although she came close. She certainly said enough to have made it clear where her priorities lay and what was most important to her. I learnt about what had happened before she came into hospital from the GP. Although we never talked about it openly, I'm convinced that she knew that I was aware of her conversations with him on the subject of dying.

During her stay in hospital, with bed rest and diuretic therapy, her condition improved substantially and after a while she was able to move around a bit and to care for herself. We discussed her future and our feeling that she really needed to enter full time care. After lengthy discussions she agreed to try a nursing home. Luckily, she had a bit of money, so it was possible to find a place for her in one of the better nursing homes.

She left the hospital on a Wednesday morning and was taken straight to the nursing home by taxi. We'd made elaborate arrangements for her sister and niece to go to her house and get whatever things she needed; she was going to try out the nursing home for a few weeks and, if she liked it, she would eventually sell or rent out her house to pay the bills.

However, the very next morning, Thursday morning, I received a phone call from the Sister-in-Charge at the nursing home. Miss T. had been at the place for less than twenty-four hours and, sick and debilitated as she was, she was out in the street hailing a taxi. I think that this gives a good indication of her personality and of her sheer strength of will. When I spoke to her some time later she explained that the nursing home was just as she had expected: the food was terrible, the nurses and doctors condescended to her as if she was senile, and the other inhabitants were, as she put it, 'just a lot of old fogies sitting around waiting to die.'

The nursing home, it seems, wasn't for her. She caught the taxi not to her own home but to her sister's place. And there they stayed together for some months. I forget how long it was – maybe two or three months. I never visited them at home, but I have a vivid mental image of what must have happened: the two elderly women, each almost as debilitated as the other, one very obese and hardly able to get about herself and the other terribly deformed and gasping for breath, grappling to get each other dressed or to the toilet. It must have been an amazing sight; it was also an indication of the spirit and mutual commitment of the two sisters.

Anyway, they managed like this for some months. During this time, Miss T. continued to attend hospital Outpatients on a regular basis. She would be wheeled in in a wheelchair by her sister or a nurse and we would discuss her medications. Her pride at having escaped the nursing home was evident.

A: Was she compliant with her medications?

PK: Yes, indeed. She was a model patient. Her medical condition was more or less stable for a time. Then one day, just at the end of the consultation, exactly as she was about to leave the consulting room, she said, 'Oh, Doctor, there's just one more thing . . . '

C: That means trouble . . .

PK: Yes, when you hear this at the end of a clinical consultation your heart usually sinks, especially if you're in a hurry, because you know that something important is about to emerge. In any case, as you can imagine, appointments with Miss T. always took longer than those with other patients.

'Yes,' I said.

'This morning, whilst washing, I noticed something in my breast. Would you mind having a look at it?'

I helped her on to the couch again and undressed her. I examined her breasts and found a lump in the right breast that seemed to me clinically to be very likely to be a carcinoma. What should I do?

B: Tell her, of course.

PK: Tell her what?

B: That you think it is a cancer. I can't see the problem.

PK: But I don't know yet that that is what it is. It is only my clinical suspicion.

B: Then say that to her. Say that you need to do some tests to confirm it.

PK: Do I need to do tests? Would that make a difference?

B: Give her the option. Say something like 'I can't be absolutely sure yet, but I think that you might have a cancer. We need to do some tests to confirm it.'

F: She wanted to die not long ago. She now has a condition that could help her die. Why not just leave it?

E: But has she said she wants to die? It seems to me that she's going pretty well at her sister's and that dying's no longer an issue.

A: But her condition's going to get worse soon. If she was that sick when she came into hospital it's only a matter of time. It might be better to bring the subject up with her again.

PK: But she hasn't said *to me* that wants to die. Should I raise the issue with her? What do you suggest? Perhaps I could introduce the subject by saying something like 'Remember once you wanted to die ... ?'

G: Look, I think this discussion is a waste of time! Why don't we talk about something important? All you need to do is use your communication skills. I came here to discuss ethics, not the irrelevant things doctors say to patients.

PK: I'm sorry to offend you, G, but I think we *are* talking about ethics. We're talking about what you actually do in face to face situations that require decisions about issues of value. Can you tell us what you would say to Miss T.?

G: You just talk to her and you tell her what the facts are. I can't see what the problem is.

PK: Perhaps we can pretend that I'm the patient at this point in the consultation. What are the exact words you'd use, G?

(Pause)

C: What did you say to her?

PK: Well, as far as I can remember, I said something like 'Yes, I can feel the lump and I am concerned about it. We could do some tests if you wish. What do you want me to do?' That seems ideologically sound, doesn't it?

She said, 'What do you recommend?'

In fact, she said this often. Although she was a strong, vivid and opinionated character – perhaps excessively opinionated – she was extremely meticulous about following any advice I would give; sometimes, this was to the point where it was embarrassing to me. She would say, 'Tell me what to do. *You* are the doctor. *I* know nothing about medicine; *my* field is English literature.' She thought this was rather a witty line and repeated it often.

A: That happens all the time. Patients always ask doctors to tell them what to do. They don't want a medical textbook; they want a prescription.

C: I agree with that. People come to doctors for advice and help about the things that doctors are good at. They trust them and do what they say.

E: But it's not as simple as that, as this very case shows. It's not just a matter of technical decision-making. The technical decisions can't be separated from the questions of life and death, the questions of a personal and maybe spiritual kind, that the doctor has no business interfering in.

D: Could you give those of us who are not familiar with this area a bit of information? What *are* the options here?

PK: Under normal circumstances, I think, the procedure would be to confirm the diagnosis with some kind of biopsy procedure. If a carcinoma were proven in this age group it would normally be removed. Often a segmental removal of the lump would be enough, although sometimes a total mastectomy is still done. The woman would then have some additional therapy – regional X-ray therapy, perhaps (although I wouldn't been keen on that here because of her underlying lung condition) and then an anti-oestrogen hormone called tamoxifen.

A: She would be a very bad anaesthetic risk. An operation would probably kill her.

PK: That's a reasonable point, but a lumpectomy could be done with regional anaesthesia.

D: What would happen if you did nothing?

PK: There are several possibilities. The tumour – if that's what it is – could remain quiescent, or, at least, it might not progress faster than her other diseases.

C: It could develop locally – it could ulcerate and fungate.

F: I've seen that. It's painful, ugly and smelly – very distressing for the patient. I wouldn't want that.

C: Or it could spread to other parts of her body – bones, brain, liver and so on.

D: You have to remove it. You can't just leave it to grow. That sounds awful.

A: You can't do anything unless you know what it is. You have to establish the diagnosis. You have to 'recommend' a biopsy first up.

PK: All right. In fact, I did that. Fine-needle aspiration cytology (where you suck a few cells up into a syringe and look at them through the microscope) was unmistakeable. It's sometimes unreliable, but here it was clear: she had an aggressive carcinoma. What now?

B: I think you should raise with her the question of dying.

E: She hasn't brought it up. You can't introduce it yourself. You can't say 'I know that you wanted to die once. Well, there's a good opportunity now!'

PK: It's true that in none of the time I knew her did she ever say to me explicitly 'I want to die'. As I said before, she came close. On one occasion, when she seemed a bit depressed, she was contemplating the end of her life. She said, quoting, I think, from Shakespeare, 'It's silliness to live when to live is torment; we have a prescription to die when death is our physician.' I waited for her to go on, but she said no more, and the subject never came up again.

F: What happened? What did you recommend?

PK: Because of the possibility of local spread and the pain and discomfort associated with that, I told her that I thought we should remove it and she readily agreed. The operation was conducted with a regional block – that is, without a general anaesthetic – and was uneventful. Pathology confirmed an infiltrating intraductal carcinoma. She was placed on tamoxifen therapy.

A: How did the wound heal?

PK: It healed well. She continued to attend Outpatients and she continued to live with her sister. I really don't know how they managed, but they did.

One day, not long after the operation she was clearly unwell and she complained that her cough was worse than usual and productive of thick, green sputum. On examination, she had a fever, but in view of her underlying chest disease it was very difficult to tell for certain whether there was any acute infection; nonetheless, clinically, I felt that there was evidence that she had pneumonia. What should I do?

G: Here we go again! I can't take any more of this! All you need to do is ask her. She is a grown woman. She knows what she wants. Just give her the facts and let her decide for herself. The trouble with doctors is that they can't believe that their clients are autonomous human beings. It's all just a power trip!

(G gets up and leaves noisily.)

PK: *(After a pause)* I think I must have said something wrong! Perhaps we should go on ...

F: You could say something like: 'I think you have pneumonia. This is an infection of the lungs. If we give you antibiotics it would probably get better. What do you want to do?'

PK: Then, knowing her, Miss T. would reply: 'What do you recommend? My field's English literature, not medicine!'

B: Then you'd have to discuss the implications of the various alternatives.

PK: Well what are they? If she has pneumonia, she may well die ...

E: I don't think she really wants to die. She's never said to you directly that she wants to die. She's just gone through an operation to remove a breast cancer. She always takes her medications. That's not the behaviour of someone who wants to die ...

B: Maybe she just doesn't want to suffer, as she said.

E: Let me finish. The only evidence that we have that she ever wanted to die was secondhand from her GP. She's gone through an awful lot since then. Who knows – maybe her life is richer and more satisfying than it's ever been before?

D: I agree with that. If she wanted to kill herself she could have done it herself months ago. She's intelligent enough. She could have taken all her pills at once or she could have found out what else she could do.

B: Would she need to come into hospital for antibiotic therapy?

PK: That would be one way of doing it – and the most effective. Alternatively, she could be given a course of oral antibiotics to take at home, with the option of a hospital admission later if desired.

B: Let's do that! If she doesn't want to take them she doesn't have to.

PK: Thanks for that – in fact, that's exactly what we did. We gave her oral antibiotics and the infection cleared. It has to be said, of course, that the clinical assessment was difficult and it is hard to say exactly what was going on. Anyway, the infection resolved.

It was about two months later that the final, tragic chapter began. It was late at night. I was off duty at the time. Apparently, Miss T.'s sister came into her bedroom to ask if she wanted some Milo before going to sleep and found her on the floor, fitting. She called an ambulance which took her straight to hospital.

She was seen in Casualty by the intern and the registrar on duty and was noted to be in 'status epilepticus' (that means she was having constant fits). For some reason (without any reference to the treating doctors) she was immediately sent upstairs for a CT scan and then to the ward. The scan showed unequivocally that she had several large space-occupying lesions in her head – almost certainly due to secondary spread of the breast cancer. She was given an intravenous drip, a nasogastric tube (that is, a tube through her nose extending down into her stomach) and anticonvulsant medications were commenced. *(Some groans and gasps are heard.)*

When I saw her the next morning her condition was essentially as I've described. She was lying in bed with intravenous and nasogastric tubes. She was drifting in and out of consciousness with frequent, barely clinical fits. From time to time, she would recognise me – enough to allow her to squeeze my hand in recognition, but she was unable to talk and certainly couldn't have a conversation.

What should we do now?

B: Let her die. Let her die. Now is the time to let her die!

D: But how? Would *you* kill her? Would you really do it?

E: Is she in pain?

PK: There is no evidence that she is experiencing physical pain.

B: She's probably suffering psychological pain. You could still give her enough morphine to kill her.

PK: Morphine in sufficient doses would certainly kill her. However, opiates also have the property of reducing the fitting threshold, so that they might actually exacerbate the tendency to fit.

F: Perhaps you could stop all her drugs. What would happen if you did that?

PK: It's always difficult to predict with certainty. Her main drugs are to control cardiac failure. It is possible that she would develop pulmonary oedema – that is, her lungs would fill up with fluid.

D: That's terribly distressing. You can't let her drown.

PK: I am interested to know what people think. Should we stop any or all of her treatment?

A: I'd stop the dig(oxin) and the Lasix (diuretic) and treat her symptomatically if she becomes distressed.

PK: What about her anticonvulsant medication?

A: No. Of course you should continue that. Convulsing would be extremely upsetting for her.

PK: What about her intravenous drip and the nasogastric tube?

A: I can't see any reason for an IV. In my unit we can almost manage without an IV. We'd usually maintain a fine-bore nasogastric for giving drugs and fluids if necessary.

PK: Well what about that question? Should she be given food and fluids?

E: She has to have 'reasonable provision of food and water'. You can't starve someone to death.

D: I've heard that it's very painful to die of dehydration.

A: That's not necessarily so. Anyway, if you need to, you can either give water through the tube or saline subcutaneously from time to time. We do that all the time.

C: I would give fluids but not food.

B: That's illogical. If you're going to feed her you should do so properly. If you want her to die you should do the job quickly!

C: But what would *you* do? Would you kill her? I couldn't do that. I could stop giving her drugs and maybe not even feed her, but I couldn't kill her.

F: Can she say anything now? Can you ask her what she wants?

PK: No, unfortunately. It's definitely too late. There's no question that she's unable to give a coherent response to any question now. Signs of recognition – a squeeze of the hand, a weak smile – are all she is capable of. I should add that there was no 'Refusal of Treatment' certificate and no Enduring Power of Attorney. I'm not sure that they would have made any difference, but all this happened before the advent of the Victorian *Medical Treatment Act 1988*.

E: It's not necessary anyway. We've had plenty of opportunities to find out from her what she wants. And in any case, what someone says under great duress can't be accepted.

PK: We'd better settle it. Who thinks that we should feed her – that is, give her food? Only one person. Who thinks that we should give her water or fluids? Most.

Well, I'll tell you what happened. We removed her drip and kept the nasogastric tube, mainly for the purpose of giving her the anticonvulsants. We stopped the medications for her heart failure – that is, the digoxin, the diuretic and the ACE inhibitor – as has been suggested. We didn't give regular fluids: that was partly because her sister and niece spent a lot of time offering food and drink to her. In fact, the two of them maintained a vigil beside her bed, giving her spoonfuls of soup whenever she would take it. It was extremely moving: they were there almost all the time – certainly, every time I came to see her, one of them was there.

Time passed – about two months, I think. Virtually nothing changed. She continued to drift in and out of consciousness and to have multiple, small fits. Her sister and her niece remained at her side, giving the spoonfuls of soup. At the end of that time she was skin and bones.

Then one day, her niece came up to me. She was very upset.

She said: 'This is just terrible! It can't go on. It is the worst of all possible worlds. It represents everything that my aunt never wanted. It's hell for her and it's hell for us!

'Do something!'

What are you going to do now?

Rodney Syme

From Innocent to Advocate: A Doctor's Path to Voluntary Euthanasia

My medical training in the 1950s did not lead me to imagine that there were areas of uncertainty in medicine. We were taught the facts, such as they were at the time, and the volume of facts to be consumed left little time for discussion of controversy and uncertainty. The explosion of medical knowledge in the forty years since then makes the idea of producing a fully fledged doctor in six years of training an impossibility. Medical ethics consisted of one lecture, which certainly did not broach a difficult matter such as euthanasia, a concept I did not encounter for some years.

I graduated in 1959, entering a medical world where paternalism was the rule. Patients were told what was wrong with them and what treatment was needed. Most practitioners did not discuss treatment options in any detail, or seek patients' opinions, or listen carefully

Rodney Syme was born in Melbourne in 1935. He graduated in Medicine in 1959, subsequently specialising in urology. He has appointments at the Austin and Repatriation hospitals in Melbourne, and a wide experience in treating cancer patients and patients with spinal injuries. He has been actively involved in the voluntary euthanasia debate since 1987, and has had articles on this topic published in the *Medical Journal of Australia* and other medical journals.

to them if they were offered. Doctors did not like their opinions being questioned. Teaching largely trained us to see problems as black or white, and carried the implication that patients always required treatment. It took me years to appreciate the possibility that some patients might simply wish to know what their symptoms meant, and that, armed with that information, they might not wish to have treatment, particularly when its invasive or potentially complicated and non-curative nature was explained to them. The prevailing medical attitude of that time has been likened to a conspiracy, though in my view an unconscious one, by Ivan Illich, whose book, *Medical Nemesis*[1], was an important criticism of the organisation and practice of modern medicine, and helped to clarify much of my own unease when I read it in the mid-1970s.

People may form views on certain subjects simply by reading extensively about them, but more often clarity comes from first-hand experience. My own path from an innocent to a determined advocate of voluntary euthanasia has been a gradual process of realisation, but with certain seminal experiences along the way. These revelations led to a greater certainty and understanding, and I think are worth sharing.[2]

In England, in 1965, during my surgical training I was called to attend an 85-year-old woman who had been struck by a car. She was deeply unconscious with obviously severe head injuries, was shocked, had a fractured leg and probable abdominal injuries. As I got into gear to resuscitate her and investigate the extent of her injuries, the soft hand of my Senior Registrar, an experienced surgeon in his late forties, restrained me, and he quietly said: 'Don't bother, son,' and went on to point out that the woman's injuries were almost certainly fatal, no matter what was done. Moreover, if she was successfully resuscitated, months of uncertain treatment would only lead to a life of total social and medical dependence, which would be an intolerable burden to her, if she were unfortunate enough to be aware of it, and to her family even if she were not. While this episode has nothing to do with 'willing to listen – wanting to die', it has much to do with the concepts of medical futility, withholding treatment, and quality-of-life issues at the end of life. It was an important first lesson regarding the conflict between quantity and quality of life.

Later that year, in another hospital, a 40-year-old man was severely jaundiced owing to gall stones. An operation to remove the stones failed and the obstructed bile duct system became infected (cholangitis). Coagulation problems developed and he became gravely ill with septicaemia (blood poisoning) and shock. I was the responsible registrar and had as my junior a 38-year-old Pakistani doctor. I told him to begin resuscitation with blood transfusion, intravenous antibiotics and anticoagulation measures. He virtually refused to take any action, stating that it was a waste of time, that the man would die no matter what treatment he was given. I did not agree and fought valiantly to save him, but the junior doctor's assessment proved correct.

I have often wondered whether this doctor's attitude was affected by his Muslim faith, which sometimes incorporates a rather fatalistic approach towards life. I did not then, and do not now agree with his attitude in this situation. It was quite clear that this 40-year-old father did not want to die, and expected everything possible to be done for him. He was capable of recovering completely with more effective treatment, and the argument that medical treatment was medically futile was not therefore tenable.

My subsequent discussion with the doctor revealed that his approach was indeed based on a fatalistic philosophy according to which 'God's Will' would be done. This episode convinced me that the doctor's religious philosophy or ethic should not intrude on the medical decision, either to continue or to withdraw treatment, and was irrelevant – it was the patient's view that was paramount and that must be sought and listened to. But the episode was a further stimulating example of an alternative philosophy to that of rendering all possible treatment in every conceivable situation. It made me think that there might be other issues involved in the care of patients.

In 1972, I treated a 52-year-old woman with kidney cancer by removing her kidney. Regrettably the cancer recurred in the spine, causing severe neuralgic pain due to pressure on nerve roots. Unfortunately, there is no effective treatment for kidney cancer, whether in the kidney or the spine, except surgery which had failed. Neither radiotherapy nor surgical exploration of the spine to relieve nerve pressure was successful in alleviating her pain. Her spine partially collapsed and her legs were partially paralysed, as was her bladder. She was in constant pain, which became excruciating every time the nurses moved or turned her. She was totally dependent on her nurse, and her quality of life was abysmal.

This combination of bone and neuralgic pain is extraordinarily difficult to treat. Blocking or dividing the affected nerves is the most effective treatment, but in this case it would have involved a major operation to divide pain fibres in the spinal cord above the cancer, leading to complete loss of sensation in the lower half of the body, a horrific procedure for a patient with a very short life expectancy. In reality her pain could only be relieved by doses of opiate analgesics or anaesthetics, which would render her comatose, and would rapidly have been fatal. She was an example of those fortunately rare cases where relief from extreme pain can only come through death.

I ordered large doses of opiate analgesics, to be given frequently. I found that the nurses were most reluctant to give these doses, for fear of the law, through allegations that they had caused, hastened, or contributed to the woman's death. In these situations it only takes one person of a certain religious persuasion to make a formal complaint and frightening consequences ensue for all. I now realise that the doctor must not only take responsibility for ordering the large doses of analgesics, but also take the lead in administering the injections whenever that is possible, in order to protect the nurses, and to encourage them to follow. Now, twenty years later, a more liberal medical policy exists regarding the use of drugs in this manner, but many doctors and nurses are still inhibited, by fear of the law, from providing adequate pain relief to the dying.

This woman's agony was extreme. For one month I visited her daily, and had nothing to offer, except to exhort the nurses to be more liberal with the analgesics. The sense of helplessness, impotence, shame and guilt that accompanied me on these visits left me in a state of considerable anguish which, however, was insignificant besides the woman's emotional and physical anguish and that of her family. My emotions also acted as an enormous block to developing a dialogue. The woman's husband asked me if there was not something more that could be done. She herself did not ever directly ask me to help end her life – had she done so, I would no doubt have sought refuge behind the law, which prevented such action and still does. I say 'sought refuge', because I fervently felt that such a request would have been totally justified and reasonable, and that to refuse that help would be morally reprehensible and cowardly. I felt helpless and impotent because the law thwarted my rendering even minimally effective assistance, shame because a society which would not allow a dog to suffer such pain did require a sentient human being to do so, and guilt because I had a sense that my own cowardice was condemning this woman to intolerable distress. Eventually her husband asked to have her moved to a hospital closer to their home, a request with which I readily agreed.

Nothing in my training or experience had prepared me for this ordeal. Hopefully one learns from such experiences and I would manage such a situation differently today. Listening is an acquired art for doctors who are more accustomed to telling. Besides, the opportunity to listen often only comes through being ready to start a dialogue after picking up the 'vibes' that patients send. In a general medical and legal climate that is antagonistic to such dialogue, it is rare for patients to directly approach their doctor with requests for help. They find it embarrassing or know it may embarrass the doctor, so they send indirect signals. Good listening therefore necessitates being open to these signals, but more importantly sending one's own signals in appropriate situations to allow a dialogue to begin. Once begun, specific counselling with unequivocal explanation of the medical situation is followed by sensitive discussion of the patient's (and the immediate family's) attitudes to relief of pain in relation to the prolongation of life.

I now know that these situations cannot be fudged, the issue cannot be avoided, the gloves must come off, and the bullet must be bitten. These are intensely challenging discussions at first, commonly avoided by doctors who have no such training, but like all things, become easier with experience. The rapport that can be established with a patient through such honest discussion is thoroughly rewarding to doctor and patient. It is rare to find a patient who is not grateful and relieved by such a discussion and thankful that he or she will retain control of the dying process and be treated with dignity and compassion.

Two years later, I was treating a 75-year-old widower with inoperable bladder cancer. Radiotherapy had helped a little, but he now had a small-capacity painful bladder; he needed to urinate every twenty to thirty minutes, with pain. He experienced severe pain in the act, and less severe pain between the acts, and incontinence if a toilet was not close by. He usually bled with each urination. The bleeding often resulted in the formation of clots, preventing urination, causing grotesque pain and leading to anaemia. No wonder generations of doctors have been taught the maxim: 'Dear God, please do not take me through my bladder.'

This man had been admitted to hospital on several occasions over a three-month period for bladder washouts to remove clots, chemical treatments via catheters to try and minimise the bleeding and transfusions to correct his recurring anaemia. Ironically, the transfusions simply prolonged his life, to go through a further cycle of futile palliative 'treatment'.

Good pain relief is possible for low to moderate pain of more or less constant intensity, but is far less effective for the sudden very severe intermittent pain that this patient was suffering. He visited me in the outpatient clinic and told me again of his extreme distress, his difficulty in urinating owing to clots, and his extreme weakness owing to anaemia. Reluctantly I told him he would have to come into hospital for bladder irrigation and transfusion. His already distressed face went paler and he shrank in his seat. 'Isn't there anything else you can do for me?' he asked. On the spur of the moment, but urged on, no doubt by cumulative experience, I recognised his *cri de coeur* and said: 'I can prescribe some sleeping tablets which you can take and you will go to sleep.' The look of relief which crossed his face is etched in my memory. It was as though an enormous burden was lifted from his shoulders. He accepted my prescription with thanks and that afternoon took all the medication.

It was actually a naive act on my part because I had never considered previously what dose of what medication would be necessary for such a patient to be successful in suicide, for that is what he wanted, and that was my intention in prescribing the medication. It was far from an ideal act of medically assisted dying and did not fulfil what I now believe, after very considerable thought and discussion, are the appropriate criteria for physician-assisted suicide. In the event, the dose was not adequate for rapid death. The man became unconscious and was found by his daughter (whom he had not told of his intention) and was brought to the hospital, resuscitated, but mercifully died of pneumonia, which was actively treated, five days later.

I was questioned by the police as to the reason for my prescription and had to lie to prevent further enquiry – and, as I only subsequently realised, the possibility of fourteen years' imprisonment for assisting suicide.

People might think I acted somewhat hastily in this case. In a sense it was because before that particular consultation I had not considered such an action. I had formed a close relationship with this man over six months and knew and understood his appalling suffering. What was sudden was my recognition of his cry for help, which was undoubtedly correct, as he took all the medication that very day. My decision to help was sudden; but it was supported by the experiences I have related, and by others. The consultation was brief, simply because I knew it was right, but also because the outpatients' department of a public hospital is not the sort of place to conduct discussions which break the law and carry a heavy penalty. I relish neither breaking the law, nor lying to protect myself, but when a cruel law punishes innocent patients, there is to me no other option.

These events taught me several things. Firstly, that patients' requests for help are only rarely direct, but more often oblique; they made me realise in retrospect that my kidney cancer patient had also asked for release. Secondly, that the law in these matters is harsh and threatening and cannot be taken lightly. I have endeavoured since then to see it changed. Thirdly, that ensuring effective suicide by a patient requires much thought, preparation and effective counselling on the doctor's part.

My own father developed pancreatic cancer in 1974; this is a particularly vicious cancer which is rarely treatable and often extremely painful. He was indeed fortunate to have his pain relieved by a visceral nerve block. His painless death was due to jaundice and gradually progressive weight loss and weakness. The calm acceptance of his fate, the equanimity with which he dealt with the situation, and the socially productive way in which he spent his remaining life had a profound effect on me and a great influence on my medical management of dying patients.

Integral to my father's ability to live positively until his death were his medical knowledge and his confidence that the particular medical environment which surrounded him would ensure that he would not suffer in a prolonged and undignified way. His medical knowledge meant that he understood his diagnosis, his prognosis, and his probable clinical course. This taught me the very great importance of giving patients the information to allow them to understand their illness, to allow them to have a measure of control in the decisions ahead of them. Acceptance of one's fate allows one to utilise the time that remains as usefully as possible. My father rejected palliative surgery, which could not prolong his life, preferring to spend that time at home doing his own thing, rather than in hospital as a medical pawn.

He was able to see and talk at length to all his friends. There are many things one might not say in everyday conversation, which one might wish to say to relatives and friends before making a final exit. In my own case, I knew when I would be seeing my father for the last time – I was able to thank him for his example to me of how a life should be used, and for the inspiration of his presence. I cherish that final conversation – we had the opportunity to say goodbye. He died peacefully at home, having accomplished all those final goodbyes that he set store by.

I do not know if he was assisted in death, nor does it matter to me. What matters is that he had a good death. That is what we would all wish for, and mercifully many of us do have a good death, without assistance. Direct medical assistance at the end of life becomes relevant only if there is uncontrollable suffering, to achieve death with dignity.

Catholics argue that it is ethically correct to administer opiates to relieve pain in terminal disease even though this might hasten death, provided the intention is to relieve pain and not to kill. Along very similar lines, I could argue that my intention in acceding to a patient's request for voluntary euthanasia is to relieve the patient's suffering and distress, which can only be fully relieved by death, which the patient wishes.

In 1976, a close relative became terminally ill with heart failure. I had known him and his wife for many years and had operated on his son. His own father had died in a protracted and undignified manner from cancer. In the course of many discussions about terminal illness, we talked not just of the matter of unrelieved pain, but of questions of loss of control of bowels and bladder, uncontrolled nausea and vomiting, extreme shortness of breath with protracted cough-ing, loss of the use of arms, legs and speech, and of a general state of distress which can be intolerable. He made much of the impact of a long terminal illness on spouse and family, who although they do not wish to lose their husband and father undoubtedly may suffer mightily in the process. I knew his feelings exactly and had a 'contract' with him that if it were possible, I would ensure that he would die with dignity.

My relative eventually entered hospital with irreversible congestive heart failure and was suffering the most distressing breathlessness. I had established from his treating physician that he was terminally ill and not responding to treatment. When I visited him, he asked me, between laboured breaths, to help him. His suffering was extreme. I asked the nurse looking after him to prepare the morphine injection which was ordered for him, and I administered it intravenously. His relief was rapid, his breathing eased, his consciousness dulled, and he died peacefully within two hours. He would have died within hours or days without that injection, but it produced the peaceful end he and his family desperately wished for.

My conscience felt clear. As far as I was concerned my commitment to voluntary euthanasia was now complete and irrevocable. But I also knew that my conscience could not remain clear unless I did all that I could to ensure that this benefit would be available to others who needed and desired it.

By 1976 I had arrived at the position that the patient's autonomy, provided he or she is rational, is paramount regarding decisions of ending life in the face of extreme suffering. I had reached this position by way of a natural experiential path; that is, I had reached this conclusion based on my own observations of medical practice and human behaviour, rather than by absorbing the wisdom of the voluminous writings on the ethical and moral arguments for and against medically assisted suicide or voluntary euthanasia. That experience told me that there was unrelieved suffering despite the best palliative care, that there were patients of sound mind who wished to voluntarily end their lives to relieve their suffering, that quality of life can be more important in terminal illness than quantity of life, and that the relief of anxiety and the provision of control to patients in the dying process is of vital importance.

Since 1976, I have studied the debate on the subject of voluntary euthanasia and refined my views on the necessary legal change. That the law needs change is beyond debate – the public clearly wishes it, and substantial numbers of doctors and nurses agree and already practise limited voluntary euthanasia at significant risk.

Three interrelated ideas impress me greatly in discussions of change. Firstly, if patients wish to end their lives because of great suffering, then that is essentially their moral right and their responsibility; secondly, that the process involving the voluntary termination of life must be such that it cannot be abused; and, thirdly, that the doctor's role in this regard should very closely resemble his or her normal mode of practice. This leads me strongly to the position of medical assistance in suicide, which allows physically and mentally competent terminally ill and suffering patients to end their lives with dignity. Medical assistance in suicide means that the doctor assists patients with advice, and through the prescription of drugs, enables them to end their lives in a dignified way. This involves the doctor in dialogue to inform the patients of their diagnosis, prognosis and treatment options. It involves ensuring that suffering in each case is significant and unalterable, that the patient is rational and not under duress, and that the request is sound and enduring. These are all medical processes of the highest order. If the doctor is satisfied beyond reasonable doubt of the *bona fides* of the request, then she or he should be able, after confirmation of the facts by a second doctor, to proceed to assistance without threat of legal sanction.

At present a doctor cannot lawfully assist a patient to commit suicide, which virtually shuts the door on any dialogue at all. Neither the patient nor the doctor can legally discuss the matter. No listening can occur, for hearing is dangerous; and if it does occur, no advice can be offered.

If the law were changed to safeguard the doctor, true dialogue could begin, and patients could clearly establish their diagnosis, prognosis, treatment options, including assistance in suicide, and the attitude of their doctor to such assistance.

The doctor could contract to give the patient honest caring support and treatment for as long as the patient requests it, but the patient knows that if the going gets too tough, help is at hand. This strong doctor-patient relationship would give control to the patient, with the doctor acting as advocate for the patient. Fear of the dying process would be relieved to allow living in dying. To a large extent control of the time, place and circumstances of death would be in the patient's control. Nothing could occur without the patient's direct intervention. The patient would be the last link in the process, rendering abuse virtually impossible. It would be the patient who has control and the final responsibility. The doctor's role would be to advise, inform, support and eventually, if necessary, prescribe the fatal medication. I envisage that the doctor would oversee the final act (but in an unobtrusive way), being aware of its timing and available to attend if necessary. If the responsibility for the final act remains in the control of the patient, then that action – as the clearest expression of 'wanting to die' – is the culmination of the doctor's 'willingness to listen'.

In the early 1990s, I was telephoned by the daughter of a 50-year-old man who was seeking assistance for her father to end his life. She told me her father had a chronic and progressive neurological disease, which had caused him to become totally dependent, with paralysis of three limbs, limited use of one arm, legal blindness, and speech difficulties. He had no bowel or bladder control and was permanently catheterised. Two years before, he had attempted to end his life, with his wife's agreement, by swallowing a large quantity of heroin tablets, and had indeed become unconscious. When, some hours later, he had not died his wife panicked and called the local doctor. A young locum attended, who agreed not to initiate resuscitation, but the patient was then taken to the local public hospital. His wife was his agent, holding a Medical Power of Attorney under the Victorian *Medical Treatment Act 1990*, and she indicated that her husband did not wish to be resuscitated. Despite this, he was resuscitated, and after further interrogation by the Public Advocate (his wife claims he was still under the influence of the drug and did not subsequently have any recollection of having given consent), a tracheostomy was performed and antibiotics were administered. As a consequence and after three weeks in hospital, the man survived but had suffered further speech impairment. The remaining function in his right arm was now deteriorating and he was becoming desperate at the thought of becoming totally dependent. His local doctor, whilst providing him with otherwise excellent medical care, was totally unsympathetic to his wish to die, and indicated that he must learn to adapt to his situation!

I was stunned by his story, and appalled by the so-called medical treatment he had received. I was appalled by the cruel and illegal manner in which his right to refuse treatment had apparently been ignored, and by the manner in which the requirement to obtain informed consent had been abused. So much for dying with dignity in 1991 under the much vaunted *Medical Treatment Act*, specifically designed to respect and protect the patient's wishes. Such a result was not surprising because the Labor Government of the day, and the Liberal Government subsequently, have done very little to promulgate the legislation.

I advised the man through his daughter to find another local doctor, to make known his views unequivocally, and to obtain at least an assurance of sympathetic medical care, if no assurance of more specific assistance (which would be illegal) was forthcoming.

A few days later, the man rang me to tell me that he could not leave the house and he could get no other doctor to visit him. Although I knew I was heading for deep water, I was impressed by this man's courage, and by the terrible ordeal he had suffered, and was continuing to face. He had been cruelly let down by the medical profession and society, and so I decided to see him and give him what advice I could.

I visited him and his wife in their home and talked with them for about two hours. His damaged voice was a flat monotone, largely devoid of expression, but despite this, he gave me the impression of great calm, strength and determination. His wife was a quiet serious woman, some years older, who had, despite his very severe disability, done her utmost to keep him at home. It quickly became clear that he realised that if his condition deteriorated, this would become increasingly burdensome to his wife (who, he wished, should be able to enjoy some quality of life of her own), or that it might be impossible for him to remain at home. He would then be totally paralysed, blind and able to talk for short periods only, with difficulty.

This man's request for some assistance to end his life struck me as totally reasonable, and the discussion left me in no doubt that he was mentally competent. I asked if he had any regrets about his previous attempt to end his life, or was he glad that it had failed. He clearly indicated that he regretted having been resuscitated and that as a result of that experience he was fearful of making another attempt, particularly since he had no medications that he knew were reliable. He was also fearful of implicating his family, since he was so disabled, in possible criminal charges of assisting in his suicide; besides, because his remaining arm function was deteriorating, he was terrified that if he waited much longer, he would lose the ability to help himself and would be trapped in total dependence, virtually unable to communicate, for an indefinite period.

At that time, I gave them general advice about the law, about the properties of some of the drugs which he had, and agreed to do some further research on drugs; but I indicated that it was too dangerous for me to prescribe potentially lethal drugs for him. I did, however, give him a categorical assurance that if he made an attempt at a drug overdose, I would admit him to hospital under my care and would ensure that no resuscitative or life-prolonging measures would be undertaken. He agreed to make a tape recording of his previous experience and his current views, which he sent to me. It reconfirmed all my impressions.

Here was a mature, competent man, who had suffered for

years from one of humankind's cruellest diseases. Approaching the later stages of the disease, he had the courage and the responsibility to attempt to end his own life, knowing that his suffering was of a kind that no medical or palliative care could alleviate – only to find that the law and the medical profession failed to protect his autonomy, condemning him instead to prolonged mental and physical suffering. He was considerate of the impact of his illness on his wife and family, immensely grateful for their care, but determined not to become trapped in total dark and silent dependence. Yet he was denied any advice or assistance in carrying out his own reasonable wish, and was fearful of the effect of a further lonely attempt upon his family if he succeeded, or upon himself if he failed (or was prevented from being successful).

I knew I was entering deep water when I agreed to meet him. On hearing his story and thinking carefully about it, I also knew that there was no way I could reach the shallows until I had given him the help he desperately needed.

We talked again several times, and about three months from the initial contact, he rang to say his arm was becoming alarmingly weak and he intended to act. I visited him again at his home with his wife and daughter present, and again discussed all the issues. He was calmly determined to proceed, and his request for help was clearly persistent. His family supported him in his decision. He indicated that he had gained comfort from my assurance about resuscitation and advice about drugs, but his concern now was that if he waited any longer he would lose the ability to help himself. I gave him specific instructions about a combination of drugs which he had available, and which should prove fatal about forty-eight hours after ingestion, and we agreed upon a date when he would take them so that I would be available to attend him if necessary.

His wife phoned me on the evening of the day he had taken the drugs to tell me he was quite comfortable. I visited him the next morning and found him conscious, without pain. He did, however, have some fever and experienced further weakness in his arm. He was transferred to hospital and received excellent care until he became comatose and died peacefully some sixty hours after ingestion of the drugs.

I have a great respect for the law. I regret that I deliberately broke it; I would have wished for a colleague, to confirm the correctness of my actions, and I would have wished to prescribe medication that would act more rapidly, but to do either of these things would have seriously jeopardised my colleague's and my liberty.

However, I have no regret regarding this event – to have denied that man help would have been an unforgivable act of cowardice and inhumanity – an immoral act.

Is it not ironic that an animal in the same condition as that unfortunate man would be granted more compassion and dignity by our society than was this helpless human being, and others like him? Is it not time for society to listen to the anguish of those who reasonably want to die? Alas, there are none so deaf as those who will not hear.

NOTES

1. Ivan Illich, *Medical Nemesis: Limits to Medicine*, Penguin, Harmondsworth, 1977.

2. Some details in the description of cases have been altered, to protect the anonymity of those concerned.

Nicholas Tonti-Filippini

Withdrawing Ventilation at a Patient's Request

As hospital ethicist at St Vincent's Hospital, an acute-care, 600-bed public hospital, I was occasionally consulted with regard to the withdrawal of chronic ventilation, both at St Vincent's and at other Australian hospitals. Here I will recount two such cases.[1] One of these, that of John McEwan, attracted a great deal of public attention at a time when the relevant laws in the State of Victoria were under review. The case became determinative of the result of that review, and the subsequent passing of the Victorian *Medical Treatment Act 1988*.

The case of **John McEwan**, perhaps more than any other case before or after it, captured the imagination of the Victorian population, whilst at the same time posing stark moral and legal questions.[2]

In January 1985, John McEwan,

Nicholas Tonti-Filippini, born in Melbourne in 1956, is a philosopher who completed his BA and MA at Monash University. For eight years he was consultant ethicist to St Vincent's Hospital, Melbourne and Director of the hospital's Bioethics Centre. From 1990 to 1992 he was based in Canberra where he conducted the Research Office for the Australian Catholic Bishops and directed the Australian Catholic Bishops AIDS Resource and Reference Centre. He is well known for his public commentary and articles on bioethics in Australia and internationally for his publications and contributions to major conferences.

then in his late twenties, was involved in a diving accident. He had dived into the Murray River at Echuca and broken his neck. From that time on until his death some fifteen months later he suffered from quadriplegia.

Some time after he had been admitted to the Spinal Unit at the Austin Hospital in Melbourne, John was told that his condition was permanent: he would always be a quadriplegic. This meant that he would be unable to use any of his muscles from the neck down, and would be completely dependent on others for all care – for washing, feeding, evacuation of his bladder and bowels, and for turning his body, to avoid pressure sores. He also had difficulties breathing. He could breathe on his own for a few hours at a time, then needed reconnecting to a ventilator to keep him alive.

Half a year after his admission to the hospital, John expressed the wish to have the ventilator withdrawn. When his request was denied, John refused to eat and, six days later, was certified insane (which would have allowed force-feeding). When he agreed to eat again, and to take antidepressant drugs, the certificate was rescinded.

During the next few months, John occasionally refused food and medication. He also frequently expressed the wish to die by having the treatment withdrawn.[3]

Twelve months after the accident, in January 1986, John McEwan left the hospital, to be cared for at his home, where he received 24-hour nursing care and was looked after by his general practitioner and a physician, Dr Joe Toscano, who specialised in spinal injuries.

Despite the fact that he was now living at home, John continued to request withdrawal of treatment. Dr Toscano refused to accede to his request – even though a psychiatric assessment stated that John was sane and that his wish to die was a reasonable response to his circumstances.[4]

John had a number of loyal friends, who understood and supported his decision. They were intimately involved in his care, and tried to help him as much as they could.

To ensure that there would be no misunderstanding, Dr Toscano gave written instructions to John's attendants and the following note dated 3 March 1986 was displayed on John's bedroom wall:

Re John McEwan

Instructions to assistants re John's ventilation treatment:

A) As John can live independently of his ventilator for up to six hours it is important to respect John's wishes to come off the ventilator if he wishes. He may wish to temporarily come off the ventilator for his own welfare.

B) Obviously if John

1. Becomes distressed

2. Has excessive secretions

3. Becomes cyanotic (turns blue because of lack of oxygen)

4. Lapses into unconsciousness

it is important that he be 'rehooked' to the ventilator although he may have indicated otherwise. At the present time as far as the law is concerned there is no law which says that if John's life is endangered by someone else's actions (not reconnecting him to the ventilator) and he dies or sustains brain damage that you as his paid assistants are not guilty of negligence and possibly more serious charges. I can be contacted at the above number at any time if any assistant etc. has any query.

Dr Joe Toscano[5]

In an effort to make those unwilling to listen hear, John and his friends had already contacted his lawyer, the media, members of State parliament, and established contact with various people working in the areas of bioethics and the law, who they thought might be able to offer some help.

I was among those contacted by John. At his request, I visited him in January 1986 at his home. John was a Catholic. He told me that he had already discussed his situation with his parish priest. The priest, John said, had reached the conclusion that the treatment he was receiving was an 'extraordinary means', and that there was, according to Catholic moral teaching, no moral obligation to continue with such treatment.

John left a lasting impression on me. He was not only a very personable man, but also a very courageous and determined one. He had explored various ways of coping with his severe disability, but had found that none of the options available to him were satisfactory. Now he was very clear about what he wanted for himself, while showing great concern for his caregivers.

I witnessed the great discomfort John was experiencing. As a quadriplegic, John had lost control of most of the functions that those of us who are healthy take for granted. He could not even breathe on his own: a machine was inflating and deflating his lungs. He was unable to cough up any sputum and required frequent suctionings – a procedure he found very uncomfortable, to say the least. This was an overwhelming difficulty and greatly added to his suffering. This utter loss of control over one's circumstances and subjection to technology can be readily borne by some people, but others, like John, find the experience constricting and unbearable.

When I met John, he had been in his present state for twelve months, and there was no reasonable chance that his circumstances would change in the foreseeable future. This led me to the following conclusions: firstly, that John had no moral obligation to continue the burdensome treatment he was receiving (even though it was desirable that he should try to do so); and, secondly, that no one had the right to demand of him that he endure the treatment.

As I've mentioned, John – with the help of his friends – tried to make his voice heard and was very successful in directing media attention to his case. There is little doubt that public opinion was on his side. Despite all this, John was not successful in his quest to have treatment withdrawn.

He was found dead on 3 April 1986, with his respirator disconnected. His attendant reported attempting to resuscitate him after his heart arrested.[6] At a subsequent coronial inquiry, the finding was that John McEwan had died of cardio-respiratory arrest associated with central nervous system malfunction; and that his death was accidental.[7]

At the time, there was still considerable uncertainty regarding a doctor's legal responsibilities in a case such as this. Dr Joseph Toscano, the specialist physician treating John McEwan, believed that John McEwan should not have been kept alive against his will. When subsequently asked why, in the face of this belief, he nonetheless continued treatment, he said that he had received legal advice to do so: 'I had been told that I would be faced with a charge of manslaughter. I did not feel that I wanted to be a martyr at that point in time.'[8]

While the advice Dr Toscano had received rested on a plausible interpretation of the law, there is no doubt that other legal advisers might reasonably have arrived at different conclusions. One thing emerged quite clearly from this case: that the law required urgent clarification. John McEwan's doctor had apparently been willing to listen to his patient's request, but ultimately felt constrained by one possible but inconclusive interpretation of the law.

The case of **Mrs N.** was different. Those caring for her were not only willing to listen to her request, they were also willing to act on it.

Mrs N. was 45 years old, married and the mother of two teenage children. She was admitted to St Vincent's Hospital with breathing difficulties. She soon stopped breathing altogether and had to be put on a ventilator, which did her breathing for her.

Initially, the doctors thought that she might have a growth on her spine which was causing the problem. Eventually, however, the diagnosis was made that she was suffering from motor neurone disease, a terminal condition affecting the nerve connections to the muscles. The condition will eventually render the sufferer totally unable to move, to speak, and to breathe. In Mrs N.'s case, the disease affected her ability to breathe first. At one stage she was actually able to walk while having her breathing assisted by a ventilator.

While at St Vincent's, Mrs N.'s condition gradually worsened and hopes of her being able to leave the hospital with ventilator assistance diminished.

I became involved in the case when I was consulted by the nursing staff, who reported Mrs N.'s frequent wish to have the ventilator withdrawn. While this would lead to Mrs N.'s death (a decision not to be taken lightly), some of the nurses also felt that it was wrong to force life-sustaining treatment on an unwilling patient.

As hospital ethicist I did not regard it as my role to become involved in a case unless invited to do so by the patient's physician, and with the consent of the patient (or his or her family in the event that the patient was incompetent). The role of a hospital ethicist is not primarily that of patient advocate; that is the role of those who stand in a therapeutic relationship to the patient. The role of a hospital ethicist is that of a consultant.

Having been made aware of the existence of some difficulties, I approached the physician with the concerns expressed by members of the treatment team. As hospital ethicist I often acted as a facilitator of communication between members of the treating team. An ethicist can articulate a problem as an independent observer, free from the immediate pressures of the complex relationships that exist within a team of highly specialised professionals.

The physician invited me to become involved in the case, to approach the patient myself and to form my own assessment of her circumstances. He openly discussed Mrs N.'s case with me, and his own concerns in regard to her medical and nursing care. He said that there was some discrepancy between what Mrs N. had apparently said to the nurses, and what she had said to him. In discussions with him, the physician said, Mrs N. had expressed a strong preference for continued ventilation. I also learnt that Mrs N. had a reputation of being a 'difficult' patient.

In my experience and that of others, dependence on a ventilator and other forms of life-support frequently has a profound emotional impact on the patient. Faced with such difficult circumstances, patients may put emotional demands on medical and nursing staff, and those demands are readily expressed by refusal of treatment - a sure way to elicit a response.

Mrs N. had two major difficulties with the treatment. First, she had suffered respiratory failure before and experienced the terrible distress involved in not being able to breathe. She lived in fear of the machine breaking down and of once again experiencing respiratory failure. Second, she had no cough mechanism so that there was a build-up of sputum which - as in the case of John McEwan - had to be suctioned off frequently by passing a thin tube down into her windpipe. For a while she had been able to do that for herself, but as time passed she was gradually weakening and had now reached the stage where she could not easily hold the tube and needed someone else to do the suctioning for her. This is an extremely uncomfortable procedure, especially when it needs to be performed many times each day.

I met with Mrs N. at her bedside. She was able to communicate with some difficulty and we discussed her circumstances. I had no reason to believe that Mrs N.'s wish to have treatment discontinued was unreasonable under the circumstances. At Mrs N.'s request I also met with her husband, to ascertain his feelings in this matter.

Following this meeting I spoke to the treating physician, who believed that treatment should be continued. When the physician asked me for an opinion, I gave the following advice: I suggested that while he should express his view regarding the continuation of life-support, Mrs N. was, in my opinion, free to choose to have this treatment withdrawn. I also pointed out that this withdrawal of life-support need not be a particularly distressing experience for the patient. Treatment could be withdrawn in carefully managed circumstances in which the unpleasant symptoms of respiratory failure would be controlled. The proposal was that the ventilator could be slowly turned down while maintaining an adequate level of oxygen. As Mrs N. could not breathe normally on her own, the effect would be a gradual build-up of carbon dioxide in her blood, which should result in a comfortable death.

The physician offered Mrs N. the possibility of withdrawing the ventilator while managing her distress. Even though he strongly discouraged her from taking that course of action, Mrs N. requested withdrawal of treatment.

Before proceeding, several doctors and a psychiatrist were consulted, and discussions took place with Mrs N. and her husband. Mr N., not wanting to lose his partner and especially concerned for the children and their dependence on her, did not initially want his wife to discontinue treatment but ultimately supported her decision. I, too, had some further conversations with Mrs N. These convinced me that her desire to have the treatment withdrawn was genuine.

I brought the matter before the hospital ethics committee and also sought a legal opinion. In addition, I attended several formal and informal meetings with the nursing staff. I recall that after one of the meetings with the nurses who were caring for Mrs N., one of the junior nurses wept and was comforted by the Director of Nursing. No one who was engaged in Mrs N.'s care found the circumstances easy.

Two important ethical conclusions were reached: firstly, that Mrs N. had no moral obligation to endure treatment which she found extraordinarily burdensome, given her terror of machine failure and the extreme discomfort of having someone else carry out the suctioning of her trachea. Secondly, we believed that Mrs N. had a moral right to refuse medical intervention. That is to say, we were of the opinion that her doctor had no independent right to treat her without her implicit or explicit, direct or indirect assent. The psychiatrist had reached the conclusion that Mrs N. was competently and reasonably refusing the intervention, and there was no evidence of any coercion. In fact, if any pressure was being applied to Mrs N. at all, it would have been pressure to continue treatment.

Six days after Mrs N. had first been given the option of treatment withdrawal, her request was implemented. With her husband by her side, the ventilator was gradually turned down while the oxygen level was increased. Mrs N. remained conscious for six hours and, in the seventh hour, died from the effects of carbon dioxide retention. The underlying cause of death was her illness - motor neurone disease. As she was unable to breathe on her own because of the disease, the carbon dioxide could not be removed from her blood and eventually led to her death.

This happened in 1988, before the *Medical Treatment Act 1988* had been passed. We knew that this action constituted a legal challenge; we did, however, believe that it was based on sound moral principles and that it was therefore appropriate for us to proceed in the way we did.

Several weeks after Mrs N.'s death, when some details of the case had become known, we held a press conference and gave a full account of the events, withholding all identifying information at the request of the family.

No one criticised our actions. No legal challenge was made.

Two comments from that period were revealing. Firstly, at a debriefing session for the nurses who attended Mrs N., a registered nurse who had cared for her previously, but who was away when she died remarked: 'So she died because she was competent.'

The comment highlighted a point for me, and I wondered whether we would have been prepared to withdraw treatment if Mrs N. had been incompetent or psychotic. Why else did we involve a psychiatrist, other than because her competence was an important factor in respecting her decision? What would happen to a less competent, less self-assured patient?

A second comment was made by Dr Paul Gerber, a lawyer who chaired a discussion held by the Medical Defence Association some months later. When introducing me as a speaker, he referred to me as coming 'fresh from the killing fields of St Vincent's'. A similar charge was levelled at me by Ms Jana Wendt in an interview on 'A Current Affair', a national television program, when she asked: 'How do you feel about the fact that some people would consider you a murderer?'

Those of us who had been involved in the case did not feel like killers or murderers. Our consciences were clear. Mrs N., we believed, had a moral right to refuse treatment she considered excessively burdensome, and it would be wrong to continue treating her against her will. Moreover, the fact that our actions were not legally challenged vindicated our confidence that doctors do not have a legal obligation to provide life-sustaining treatment when the patient competently, freely and informedly refuses that treatment.

In many ways, the situation was unique. At that time, I was the only hospital ethicist in Australia, and we were then the only hospital in Australia with an ethics research facility. I also happened to have a very competent barrister on my staff who helped form our thinking. In addition, St Vincent's was a Catholic hospital with a strong moral tradition behind it, and we were applying the Church's clear teaching; firstly, that these decisions are to be made by the patient, and, secondly, that the patient is not obliged to make use of overly burdensome means to prolong life.

We were also able to rely on the long-established reputation of St Vincent's as morally conservative, and on the trust the community placed in the individuals concerned, whose public testimony to Catholic moral teaching was well known. I doubt that doctors, acting as we did but on their own, would have been received so well, nor would they have been so well placed to explain the course of events.

Because of these circumstances, our situation was significantly different from that faced by many other health care professionals and patients, who had to make these kinds of decisions on their own, without moral or legal guidance. There is public evidence to suggest that many other people in similar circumstances were placed in intolerable situations by the failure of the law to determine the limits of patients' rights and doctors' obligations.[9] John McEwan's case is, of course, an example of this. Doctors confronted by a competent patient refusing life-prolonging treatment were caught between a rock and a hard place, between the law of negligence (if they did not provide life-support) and the law of trespass to the person (if they were to continue treatment).

In Victoria, the issue has now been resolved through the implementation of the *Medical Treatment Act*, but it still requires resolution in the other Australian states. The *Medical Treatment Act* provides that competent patients, who are not obviously suicidal, have the right to refuse medical treatment, even life-sustaining treatment; at the same time, the *Act* gives legal protection to doctors who implement the patients' requests. Legislation of this kind is highly desirable. Respect for the patient's moral right to refuse treatment - to be listened to, if you like - should not require health care professionals to courageously jeopardise their reputations, nor should it require them to place themselves at legal risk of prosecution. At the same time, of course, any such legislation ought not to facilitate suicide or homicide.

So how do we distinguish between refusing burdensome treatment, suicide and voluntary euthanasia? Does a patient's request to have a respirator withdrawn show suicidal intent, and are doctors who accede to such a request assisting a suicide? The question is important from a moral and a legal point of view. Although suicide has been decriminalised, assisted suicide remains a crime in all Australian states, a point quite clearly stated in the Victorian *Medical Treatment Act*.[10] Also, from the Catholic point of view suicide is regarded as self-killing, and is considered absolutely wrong. This moral stance would, of course, also rule out assisted suicide or voluntary euthanasia.

In many cases it is clear when a person has committed suicide, or attempts to commit suicide. Swallowing a lethal dose of sleeping pills with the intention of ending one's life would be one example of this.[11] In such cases, it is normal practice in Australian hospitals to try and save the life of the person who has attempted to end his or her life. This practice is supported by the law. When a suicidal person is taken to a hospital, emergency treatment may be instigated without the informed consent of the patient. Urgent action is required, and the assumption is that the patient may be severely depressed or otherwise not competent.

This paternalistic approach is justified on the grounds that suicide attempts are often carried out at times when the person suffers from severe and perhaps temporary depression. Under such circumstances, the attempt may be a plea for help, rather than a genuine attempt to end one's life. There is thus reason to question the mental state of the patient, and it will often be morally and legally justifiable to provide life-sustaining treatment, even if the patient refuses it.

The problem is to distinguish suicidal refusal of the medical treatment from cases where patients such as John McEwan or Mrs N. refuse medical treatment because they regard it as excessively burdensome.

In the late 1980s the Victorian Social Development Committee conducted an inquiry into death and dying, entitled *Options for Dying with Dignity*. In its report under the same title, the Committee drew a clear distinction between suicide and voluntary euthanasia on the one hand and the refusal of treatment on the other. The Committee thus rejected the notion that patients have a 'right to die', but supported the view that patients have a right to refuse treatment – even if this will lead to their death. The right to refuse treatment under the appropriate circumstances was not, the Committee thought, the same as committing suicide and did not amount to the deliberate or intentional termination of life. As far as the deliberate ending of life was concerned, the Committee did not recommend that the law relating to assisted suicide, murder and manslaughter should be changed – changes that would be necessary if doctors were to be legally allowed to assist patients in the deliberate ending of their lives.[12]

The moral relevance of the distinction between the refusal of life-sustaining treatment and the deliberate ending of a patient's life is increasingly being challenged. Some people believe that it does not make much of a moral difference whether a doctor, at the patient's request, turns off a respirator or ends the patient's life by more direct means – for example, by prescribing a lethal dose of a drug, or by administering a lethal injection.[13] Much has been written on this point, but this is not the time to enter into what has become a rather involved and intricate debate.

In accordance with traditional Catholic thinking, I take the view that a clear moral distinction can and must be drawn between the refusal of treatment because the treatment is burdensome, and the deliberate shortening of a patient's life by withdrawing non-burdensome treatment. The deliberate shortening of human life is always morally wrong; the refusal of burdensome treatment is not.

This is not merely a matter of moral or religious respect for human life. Such a radical departure from the fundamental moral and legal tenet that all human lives are inviolable would also be fraught with great social dangers. Whilst the social provision of assisted suicide or voluntary euthanasia might enhance the liberty of some people, it would at the same time jeopardise the life and liberty of many others – the lives of those who are weak and vulnerable.

We need legal structures which will protect us against all forms of homicide. Without such structures individuals cannot live together in a community without fear.

Human life has inherent dignity. The dignity of the seriously ill can, I believe, be diminished through the inappropriate use of medical technology. By this I mean the employment of medical technology to sustain a patient's life, irrespective of the patient's beliefs, values, and own evaluation of the circumstances. The cases of John McEwan and Mrs N. illustrate this point. Mrs N. was allowed to die with dignity, John McEwan was not.

The intrinsic dignity of human life can also be diminished in a second way, namely by the judgement – inherent in voluntary euthanasia and suicide – that some lives are not worth living.

Therapeutic obstinacy, that is, keeping patients alive against their will, and voluntary euthanasia/suicide are in some respects two sides of the same coin. They are expressions of the inability to accept the dying process, diminishing function and, to a degree, suffering as a part of life. The frantic efforts to save life, in the face of the inevitable, involve the same logic and the same premise which seeks to avoid the reality of suffering by opting for suicide or voluntary euthanasia. Both approaches reflect a denial of reality and a desire to control, to exercise power over that which is, or should be, beyond human control.

In each case respect for human dignity is diminished because in each case the patient's life is sacrificed to the desire to be in control of the situation. In each case the patient is the object not the subject of his or her illness and its medical management. This is true even in cases where the patient acts with suicidal intent.

Self-destructive actions are not only an offence against human dignity; they are also an offence against the community - for the good of the community depends on respect for human life. To protect the good of the community, it is important that we have laws that discourage or prohibit self-destruction. The law ought not to endorse suicide, assisted suicide or voluntary euthanasia. The community may, of course, for practical reasons decide not to punish suicide attempts, but this must not in any way imply approval of suicide or voluntary euthanasia.

NOTES

1. A shorter and more technical account of the cases described here appeared in the *Medical Journal of Australia*, vol. 157, 17 August 1992, pp. 277–79.
2. *Court Record 4/12/86*, Coronial Enquiry into the Death of John McEwan, Melbourne Coroner's Court.
3. Evidence to the Coroner given by Mary McEwan, John's mother, ibid.
4. ibid.
5. Social Development Committee of the State Parliament of Victoria, *Inquiry into Options for Dying with Dignity, Minutes of Evidence*, 2 March 1987.
6. *Court Record 4/12/86*, Evidence of Henry Robert Thomas to the Coronial Enquiry, op.cit.
7. *Court Record 4/12/86*, Melbourne Coroner's Court, ibid.
8. Social Development Committee, *Inquiry into Options for Dying with Dignity, Minutes of Evidence*, 2 March 1987.
9. Social Development Committee, *Inquiry into Options for Dying with Dignity, Second and Final Report*, 1987, pp. 17–42.
10. *Medical Treatment Act 1988 (Vic.)*, Part 1, Section (3).
11. See the case of Graham Michael Kinney. I discuss this case in my article 'Some refusals of medical treatment which changed the law of Victoria', *Medical Journal of Australia*, vol. 157, 17 August 1992, pp. 278 ff.
12. Social Development Committee, *Inquiry Into Options for Dying with Dignity, Second and Final Report*, op.cit., v.
13. See, for example, Helga Kuhse, *The Sanctity-of-Life Doctrine in Medicine - A Critique*, Oxford University Press, Oxford, 1987.

Kenneth Ralph

At the Bedside

In the twenty-five years I have practised as a Protestant clergyman few people have asked me to help them find a way to end their lives, even though for most of that time I have been a public supporter of active voluntary euthanasia. This is not surprising. Even though three quarters of the Australian population support active voluntary euthanasia, very few people will, in the end, need it for themselves. Mother Nature is benign, to most of us. We will die gently, peacefully and without undue pain.

But from time to time, dying people do implore me to use some influence somewhere, with someone, to call a halt to what is happening to them. Perhaps they think I can persuade God or their physician or whoever, to do the right thing and put an end to what for them is an existence that no longer makes any sense.

Kenneth F. Ralph was born in 1936 in Auckland, New Zealand and is now a naturalised Australian. After completing a BA at Otago University, New Zealand, he trained as a Presbyterian minister at Princeton Theological Seminary, New Jersey, USA. He has practised as a minister of religion in America, New Zealand and Australia and is currently a minister of the Uniting Church in Australia.

He also trained in psychotherapy at Melbourne's Cairnmillar Institute, acting as a consultant for that organisation for several years. He conducts a private counselling practice in Geelong, Victoria.

I always find these requests for assistance to die most disconcerting – not because I think they ought not to be made, but because they cannot, without breaking the law, be respected and acted upon.

I started to believe in voluntary euthanasia a quarter of a century ago. It all began with Tom's two wives in my first year as a clergyman.

Tom's first wife, a member of our church, was admitted to hospital with stomach pains. Tests disclosed that she had a fast-growing, inoperable cancer. She was sent home to be treated by her local doctor. For the remaining weeks of her life, I visited her frequently, in my role as parish minister, taking with me the prayers of the church. The doctors took pain-killers. Friends took flowers. Tom's wife quickly lost weight, sank into lethargy and finally into long periods of sleep and unawareness. She lost control of her functions as well as her dignity. She died in pain.

When I officiated at her funeral, I felt helplessness, admiration for all those directly involved, sadness and a strange unease about having been an accessory to something that surely could have been prevented. Why did her dying have to go on for so long? Why was the pain not adequately reduced, or stopped altogether? What benefit was there for this woman, her husband, her family, in this seemingly endless three-month terminal phase? At the ceremony I said the words of divine love, but wondered just how loving and responsible we had really been.

Through it all Tom had kept up his courage, as is often the case in these circumstances. Despite his growing fatigue, he was an enormous support to his wife and to us all at the bedside.

Life flowed on. Within a year, Tom was engaged to a woman from his community who had been a family friend for many years. Soon they were married. But their happiness was not to last. Shortly after their marriage, she too was diagnosed as having cancer.

For Tom the second time around was terrible. His new wife was not as brave, or stoic, as his first wife had been. She did not have the same toleration of pain. She hated the deterioration of her condition – and she voiced the wish that someone would help her to end it all. Tom was different too. His physical and emotional resources were much depleted. He found himself getting cross with his wife and felt awful about it afterwards. Tom was a Presbyterian, but his faith, which had been such a support to him the first time around, no longer came to his aid. This time, he could no longer so readily accept the idea that suffering is inevitably part of some grand, albeit unfathomable, divine plan which gives it dignity and meaning.

As a clergyman and a person I was different too. A cluster of convictions had begun to evolve. One was the view that the wish to end one's life in such a situation was not necessarily bad or sinful. Another was the belief that a person's request for the termination of life needed to be taken seriously, rather than be deflected as the vocalisation of someone who was depressed, lacked faith, or was merely fearful. A third conviction was that under certain circumstances people should be able to obtain the means to end their lives, and that it should not be unlawful to assist them in this task. Lastly, it seemed to me that if there was a God, which I did not doubt, and if this God was compassionate, which seemed to me to be axiomatic, and if this God's chief concern was the welfare of the human beings He or She had so marvellously designed, then such a God would have no trouble saying 'Yes' to the request of someone like Tom's second wife.

Despite these ruminations, I continued to take the prayers to Tom's second wife; the doctor took the pills; the friends the flowers; and the beautician took the wig to make up for the hair that had fallen out.

189

At that time I had not long graduated from Princeton Theological Seminary in New Jersey, USA, where along with 500 other students I had been accustomed to hearing visiting international speakers. One of them was a pipe-smoking, Mozart-loving German theologian by the name of Karl Barth. He was famous not only for his massive religious writings, but even more so for having warned the world, in a pamphlet entitled 'Against the Tide', about the growing totalitarian menace which followed the election of Adolph Hitler in 1933.

Barth, who had a significant influence on post-war Protestant thought, was much opposed to euthanasia, as well as to abortion and suicide. The historical cultural reasons for this are not difficult to find. He had been appalled by the devaluation and trivialisation of human life under Hitler.

Barth was joined in his protest against Hitler, and on issues such as suicide, abortion and euthanasia, by a fellow clergyman by the name of Dietrich Bonhoeffer. Bonhoeffer's objection to Hitler's regime eventually led him to take part in an unsuccessful bomb plot to kill the Führer. In prison for this offence (Bonhoeffer was eventually executed), he wrote an influential book on ethics in which he attacked euthanasia.[1]

Had Barth or Bonhoeffer been at the bedside of Tom's second wife, they would no doubt have been good listeners and supportive and caring pastors. But had the woman indicated to them that she wished to be helped to die, we can be sure that these men would have done little more than reaffirm the Church's traditional prohibition of any life-shortening act.

The traditional argument against voluntary euthanasia – and the one that Barth and Bonhoeffer would undoubtedly have appealed to – is that a person's life does not belong to her- or himself, but to God, who gives it to each of us as a gift or on loan. Life, they might have said to the woman, reflects divine existence and is the most sacred of all that exists. Such a gift must be treated responsibly and with respect, and must be protected against any act that would negate or destroy it.

According to this view, then, we humans are forbidden to dispose of our own life, regardless of the situation in which we find ourselves. Barth, for example, argued that God alone decides if a life is a success or a failure, if it is tolerable or intolerable.[2] This view was endorsed by Bonhoeffer when he wrote that no matter how much of a torment our own life is to us, we must not use our freedom before God to act against it. We must not deliberately end our life; rather we must keep it intact in all circumstances, even if pain and suffering render it so utterly intolerable that death would seem a merciful release.[3]

Within a few years of the death of Tom's second wife, the seeds of doubt about this traditional position of the Church had grown full size in me. A new position was in place, one which said that voluntary euthanasia was a morally acceptable act, entirely consistent with the Christian message.

Nowadays, the conviction which says 'Yes' to such acts as voluntary euthanasia and assisted suicide in the case of the terminally and incurably ill, is regularly found in the pews of Australian Christian churches, but not often heard from its pulpits, and hardly ever endorsed in Australian ethical-pastoral writings. No mainstream church in Australia has ever endorsed voluntary euthanasia in principle or even as a right of private conscience.

Support for active voluntary euthansia at a scholarly level within the Church is mainly American. One prominent Church leader who has advocated voluntary euthanasia was the Reverend Dr Joseph Fletcher, a famous American professor of ethics whose writings have been influential in the voluntary euthanasia movement.[4] Another was the Reverend Dr Leslie Weatherhead who a long time ago declared that he was willing to give a patient Holy Communion and stay with him or her while the doctor administered the means to end the patient's life.[5] And in a dramatic way the Reverend Dr Henry Van Dusen, President of Union Theological Seminary in New York, gave credence to the voluntary euthanasia movement when, in 1975, he entered into, and executed, a suicide pact with his wife. She had suffered from severe arthritis, and he had been the victim of a stroke that left him impaired. Twenty-five years earlier, he had joined with forty other religious leaders to openly state his support for voluntary euthanasia.[6]

The Church sometimes gets criticised for its head-in-the-sand position over voluntary euthanasia. While such criticisms are richly deserved, I nonetheless believe that the Church should also be given credit for having provided from its ranks some strong leaders who have taken a contrary and more humane view. These people have not only developed some of the central ethical and theological arguments that underpin the now worldwide so-called 'right to die' movement, but they have also had the courage to go public at a time when it was not popular to do so.

Breaking away from the prohibitory morality of the past, a plausible and more humane contemporary Christian position allows terminally ill persons to end their own lives, or to request others – for example, doctors – to help them in this quest. Such an ethic requires of them solid reasons, consistent with certain rigorous ethical standards, to justify their wish to die, and assures the suffering person that a request to die can be legitimate and entirely compatible with the Christian message. What is more, for those who wish it, this contemporary Christian ethic offers to bring to the bedside the elements of Holy Communion, at the same time as the doctor brings the means that will grant the patient a final release.

Three great religious and ethical principles undergird this position. These can be invoked to facilitate decision-making at the bedside. The first principle affirms the value of human life; it asserts that each person's life has exquisite and intrinsic worth. The second principle, that of moral autonomy, requires us to respect the autonomy of others, that is, to allow other persons or moral agents to shape and determine their own destiny. And finally, the third principle, that of beneficence, asks us to act beneficently towards others, that is, to do them good rather than harm.

According to the traditional Christian view, human life has absolute value. Contemporary Christians and others frequently take a different view. They might wholeheartedly agree that life (*bios*) has intrinsic value, is beautiful, good, and exquisite, and that nothing external can diminish this inherent beauty. If they are religious, they would also affirm that there is a spiritual dimension to life, that we are imbued with divinity and that this enhances the intrinsic value or dignity of human life.

But the view that life has great intrinsic worth does not commit one to the view that life must always be sustained and that extrinsic factors – such as state of health, the desires and wants of the ill person, and so on – count for nothing. On the contrary. As wonderful and awe-inspiring as it is to have life, biological life is always only the precondition for a range of other things that give beauty and meaning to a human life.

It is not difficult to imagine situations in which being the possessor of life would be a most dubious asset. Imagine, for example, that you have had an accident and suffered brain injury, not enough to kill you, but enough to leave you in a persistent vegetative state, with a life expectancy of another twenty years. You would not know who you are, and probably not even *that* you are. Your capacities for making contact with others would be non-existent. In such a situation many people would want to say that even though they hadn't stopped being human (and their life still had intrinsic value), they now lacked too many of the important characteristics of true humanness to make life valuable for them. They would not wish to live such a life.

Some people put themselves imaginatatively into these types of situations and come to the view that if they were to lack adequate self-awareness, emotional responsiveness, the capacity to give and receive affection; if they lacked the ability to make judgments for themselves; if their communication skills were reduced to grunts, mumbles or worse; if they were not aware of time, occupancy of their own body, or of their surroundings; and if these conditions were irreversible, then they would not want to be the possessor of such a life, because it would have for them, at the most, minuscule merit and might be a great burden.

Similar arguments can be advanced in the case of terminal illness which – whilst it might leave a person's mental faculties intact – would leave her or him with nothing but pain, suffering and discomfort, and a life that is experienced as an intolerable burden. Again, it is not difficult to see why some people would not wish to live such a life.

To lack the characteristics of what makes up true (not just biological) humanness, thus provides for some people the rationale for seeking an early death. For others it is the terminal suffering, the slow (and from their point of view) undignified decline so often associated with terminal illness that justifies their wish to die. Wishing to die in such situations is not to deny the intrinsic value of human life; it is rather to say that from personal or experiential point of view life in those types of situations has little or no value to the person whose life it is.

Such assessments are subjective. In these matters there is only one truth, the truth for us. We can only make these types of assessment for ourselves. No one can make them for us, and we cannot assess the value of the life of another person.

I have thought about these matters, and so has my wife. We each know the other's view about 'the Good Life', the kind of life we would want to live and the kind of life we would find intolerable. She knows the circumstances in which I would want my life to be ended, and I have a good sense of when enough would be enough for her. Like the Van Dusens, we have pledged that we will help each other, if ever we find ourselves in a position of extremity. Some people object that this process of assessing the value of life is un-Christian because it relativises morality; throws the Ten Commandments out the window; rejects the biblical teaching on the absolute sanctity of human life; and audaciously makes individual humans, not God, the decision-makers with respect to life and death issues.

To this a contemporary Christian like myself would reply that 'absolute' is a word that cannot properly be applied to human life or to values, or even to God in the Bible. Life is a relative, not an absolute, good. In the Christian context, life is not seen as absolutely sacred, as inviolable, or as possessing absolute value. This is why the Bible does not have a universal prohibition against direct killing. It endorses war. It provides for capital punishment. It fails to condemn any of the four cases within its own pages where people commit suicide.[7] And that is why Karl Barth was not a pacifist, any more than most Christians are, and why Dietrich Bonhoeffer found a way to justify both his attempt to assassinate Hitler, and to approve of voluntary martyrdom, where a person deliberately lays down her or his life for an ideal.

Absolutising the sixth commandment has never been possible. Even those who compiled the Bible were incapable of it. If Exodus 20 gives us the famous formula which is sometimes translated: 'Thou shalt not kill'[8], it is the very next chapter which gives four grounds for killing another human being: if you strike your parents; if you kidnap someone; if you murder someone; if you curse your parents.[9]

The nearest the Bible comes to absolutising a value is when it recounts Jesus's 'great commandment', the imperative of love.[10] This love is unchanging in character, but expresses itself differently in each new situation. As an ethical code it serves us well. It carries more humaneness, elegance and is more helpful in the human context than the Ten Commandments, which it supplants and transcends. This great commandment of love is linked to the other two fundamental ethical and religious principles mentioned above – the principles of autonomy and beneficence – to which I now turn.

To love another is to respect the other as a person, as an autonomous individual who is morally entitled to lead her or his own life in accordance with her or his own values and beliefs. In the medical context, this means that the first and central question must be this: 'What does the person want for him- or herself?' What is of central importance is thus not what the doctor wants, what the patient's partner or children want, what Moses might want, or what an ecclesiastical authority or some guru of a human relations group might want. The decisive question is: 'What does the patient want?'

Autonomy or self-determination is central to what it means to be a human being or a person. It is linked to such notions as freedom and choice. There is no morality without choice and no choice without the freedom to decide between alternatives. There has to be the possibility of a judgment between A and not-A. Autonomous people make their own choices and accept the responsibility for these choices.

Christianity has always been a champion of this position. Even the early creation myth of Adam and Eve enshrines the biblical principle of personal choice and personal responsibility. Adam and Eve were created as free moral agents, who were given the capacity to make decisions for themselves. One of their first choices concerned a famous apple. Some philosophers claim that God could have created Adam and

Eve in such a way that it would have been in their nature to resist choosing the apple. Religious thinkers, however, generally take the view that this would not have constituted a situation of real choice and would thus be anathema to what it means – in the religious context – to be human. There would have been no discriminating free judgment between real alternatives, and the one who made this so-called choice would have been neither free, nor moral, nor spiritual nor human. Self-determination is thus seen as a key component in being a moral person.

Self-determination is important not only in the religious and moral context, but is also the centrepiece of the voluntary euthanasia movement. If a dying person has not *asked* to be assisted to die, then that assistance, supporters of voluntary euthanasia say, may not be provided. You have to put your hand up and say that you want it before you can have it.

Now imagine that a religious person who believes in the great commandment of love stands by the bedside of someone like Tom's second wife, who is terminally ill and ardently desires to die. For such a person, the question is this: 'How can the great commandment of love Jesus gave us be fulfilled in this concrete case? What is the most loving thing here?' This person is not thinking about love in its sentimental form but that form which seeks the well-being of the other.

While Christians call this principle, which seeks the well-being of others, 'love', secular ethicists often call it 'beneficence'. This principle, irrespective of what we choose to call it, asks us to do that which enhances the lives of others and maximises their well-being, as perceived by them.

Here we need to note that what will benefit or harm a person will vary with the circumstances. Life is normally a good thing, and doctors would therefore normally be benefiting their patients by extending their lives. But this is not always the case. If a patient is terminally ill, suffers much and wants to die, then life is no longer a benefit and death becomes a merciful release. The Protestant clergyman Joseph Fletcher calls this approach, which focuses on the particularities of the situation, 'situation ethics' or 'case ethics'. It involves choosing that course of action that will, under the circumstances, best serve the interests of those affected by our action.[11] It is a consequentialist ethics because it justifies our actions by the good consequences they produce.

If one comes to the bedside equipped with this principle of love or beneficence, and makes this particular sick and suffering person who wants to die one's moral focus point, then it is easy to see why one would sometimes come to the conclusion that an early death would benefit this person most and should be granted as an act of love. Continued life is no longer of any benefit to the person who is bearing the pain and wants to die. It is pointless, demeaning, degrading, absurd. Love's discriminating voice pronounces that enough is enough.

In some cases not only is no good being done, but actual harm is occurring when we keep a suffering person alive, against his or her will. The old medico-moral principle 'do no harm' is being violated in such cases because we are keeping a person alive in an intolerable, inhuman situation against that person's wishes. *You* may not think the situation is intolerable, but that is not the point. You are not the one who suffers, who bears the pain. You are not the one who, before becoming comatose, declared that she or he would not want to be kept alive in that state. It is not your life.

Sometimes the only way in which we can release a person from a life of suffering he or she no longer wants is by taking active steps to end that life. We take that option up with our hopelessly ill pets because greater harm is done by keeping them alive in their misery. Such actions are also morally acceptable in the human context – in situations where all else has failed and nothing more can be done; where our action will release another person who has earnestly and consistently indicated that she or he wants to die from a life of pain and suffering. To assist people in such circumstances – either by providing them with little white pills, for them to swallow by themselves, or by intervening as a third party, through the administration of a lethal drug – is, I believe, ethically acceptable.

I have no doubt that assisting human beings to die in this way is consistent with the personalist ethics of Jesus, the founder of Christianity. I look forward to the day when the civil courts of Australia will permit it for those who wish it, and when our ecclesiastical courts will endorse it as a liberty of conscience issue. Few will need it. As I said before, Mother Nature's way for most of us is benign – we will die gently, peacefully and without too much pain.

What strikes me about the people who support voluntary euthanasia is that by and large they are great celebrators of life. What they fear is degradation and unrelievable suffering. They are pro-active people, who champion the great human virtues of autonomy, faith, courage and compassion. They recognise that sometimes suffering has a benefit and purpose, but that in other cases it can be utterly meaningless and destructive.

People who support voluntary euthanasia do not see themselves as 'playing God'. The way they view it is that they are taking responsibility for their living and dying which, they believe, is something God would want them to do. They do not believe that God decides when and how we die. They say that death is a natural phenomenon. There is no need to bring God into it: it seems crude to conceive of God as the one who decides who will die this day or the next, and of this cause or of that.

For myself, I would have thought that God would be rather pleased that the ones He or She has designed had turned out to be so adventurous and sensible as to choose the voluntary euthanasia option in a time of extremity, to take the initiative, to get into the boat by themselves and launch it out across the River Jordan. And if they came singing the Gloria and reciting the Nunc Dimitus 'Now Lord let your servant depart in peace', all the better.

NOTES

1. Dietrich Bonhoeffer, *Ethics*, Macmillan, New York, 1962.

2. Karl Barth, *Church Dogmatics*, III:4, T. & T. Clark, Edinburgh, 1961, p. 404.

3. Bonhoeffer, *Ethics*, p. 125

4. Joseph Fletcher, *Humanhood: Essays in Biomedical Ethics*, Prometheus, New York, 1979; also *Moral Responsibility: Situation Ethics at Work*, Westminster Press, Philadelphia, 1977.

5. Leslie Weatherhead, *The Christian Agnostic*, Hodder & Stoughton, London, 1965.

6. Doris Portword, *Common Sense Suicide: The Final Right*, Grove Press, New York, 1978, p. 69.

7. Saul (I Samuel 31:4); Antithopel (II Samuel 17:23); Samuel (Judges 16:30); Judas (Matthew 27:5).

8. Exodus 20:13

9. Exodus 21:12–16.

10. Matthew 22:37–39.

11. Joseph Fletcher: *Situation Ethics: The New Morality*, The Westminster Press, Philadelphia, 1966.

PART THREE
Assuming Responsibility

'A good death is ... a death I choose and determine
for myself – and ... something that a liberal society
should favour and foster ... '

Max Charlesworth

A Good Death

Issues about death and dying are often considered in abstraction from the social and cultural and political context in which they arise. But it is obvious that one's view of these issues will be, or ought to be, different in a liberal society as compared with other kinds of society.

In a liberal society personal autonomy, the right to choose one's own way of life for oneself and correlative respect for the right of others to do the same, is the supreme value. Certain consequences follow from the primacy given to personal autonomy in a liberal society. First, in such a society there is a sharp disjunction between the sphere of personal morality and the sphere of the law. The law is not concerned with matters of personal morality and the 'enforcement of morals'. Second, the

Max Charlesworth is an Emeritus Professor. Formerly Professor of Philosophy and Dean of the School of Humanities at Deakin University, he has been a member of the Australian Health Ethics Committee, of the National Health and Medical Research Council, the Bioethics Committee of the Royal Australian College of Obstetricians and Gynaecologists and the Victorian Standing Review and Advisory Committee on Infertility. Currently he is Director of the National Institute for Law, Ethics and Public Affairs at Griffith University. He is the author of *Bioethics in a Liberal Society* (1993).

liberal society is characterised by ethical pluralism which allows a wide variety of ethical and religious (and non-religious) positions to be held by its members. Third, apart from the commitment to the primacy of personal autonomy and respect for the autonomy of others, there is no determinate social consensus about a set of 'core values' or a 'public morality' which it is the law's business to safeguard and promote.

If we take the liberal ideal seriously and follow it consistently, we are led to radical conclusions in many areas of medical ethics and bioethics. Thus, for example, the value of personal autonomy ought to play a central part in discussions about the limits of medical treatment, the rights of patients to refuse treatment and even in some circumstances to bring about their own deaths. In general, it means that we ought to be able to control the manner of our dying in the same way that we control the manner of our living. It follows that deliberately taking one's life is, in certain circumstances, neither immoral nor antisocial.

Again, the liberal idea of personal autonomy and self-determination is central to the discussion of the new reproductive technologies (*in vitro* fertilisation, for example) and the novel modes of birth and family formation they make possible. The principle that women have a right to control their own reproductive processes is a corollary of the principle of personal autonomy and some have spoken of a 'right to procreative liberty'. In other words, people should be free to choose their own alternative ways of having children and forming families and we ought to see the various forms of assisted procreation, as in *in vitro* fertilisation and IVF-assisted surrogacy, as means of enhancing our personal autonomy and freedom.

Finally, the debate over the just or equitable distribution of health resources in the community has so far been dominated by utilitarian, economic rationalist, cost-benefit oriented approaches which are authoritarian and bureaucratically paternalistic in style. Against this, one might argue that in a liberal society the expansion of patient choice and control of health care resources should be a major goal of any system of health care allocation.

A liberal society is one where people take up a wide variety of ethical and religious positions and where they tolerate and respect others' positions. In effect, they agree to disagree about ethical and religious issues and they do not seek to impose, by legal or other means, their ethical views on other people. It is only when other people are harmed or when their right to choose for themselves is violated in some way, that the law may intervene. This means that it is pointless to search for some kind of religious or moral 'consensus' – a commitment to a set of basic values (apart from the value of personal autonomy and respect for the autonomy of others) about which we all agree – upon which our society is founded and without which it will break apart and end in anarchy.

The liberal ideal has been sharply attacked by critics from different quarters: for example, some Christian thinkers claim that a society must make substantive value commitments – to the sanctity of human life, to traditional marriage and the family and so on; again, certain political philosophers claim that no one is really capable of the kind of autonomy and self-determination required by the protagonists of liberalism, and further that the so-called liberal society is based upon atomistic individualism which allows no scope for community life.[1]

I believe that these criticisms are misconceived and that the liberal ideal can be successfully defended against them. Here, however, I wish to focus upon certain questions about death and dying in an attempt to show how our consideration of them should reflect the values that animate a liberal society.

As I have just remarked, the notion of personal autonomy is central in any discussion of the rights of people to decide whether they should allow their lives to be prolonged or whether they may end their lives, directly or indirectly. The principle that applies here is that as autonomous moral agents we have a right and a responsibility to control the course of our lives; so also as autonomous agents we have a right and a responsibility to control when and how we die. Of course circumstances may on occasion prevent us from controlling the course of our lives and how we die, but the principle remains valid that, as far as circumstances allow, we should strive to exercise autonomous control over the way we live and the way we die.

Put in another way, we should be free as moral persons to make decisions for ourselves about whether we wish to refuse medical treatment or to have such treatment withdrawn, or to have recourse to palliative treatment (for example, by painkilling drugs) that we know will hasten our death, or even to bring about our own death by direct means or to ask for assistance from another to bring about our own death.

I might remark in parenthesis that the term 'euthanasia' is now so hopelessly compromised that it leads to confusion to use it here. An autonomously chosen death where I choose to die because I judge, for appropriate reasons, that further physical survival would be medically futile and humanly pointless, has nothing to do with the case where another person – a physician or a nurse – judges on objective medical grounds, without reference to my wishes, that my 'quality of life' is so negligible that my life should be terminated, either directly or indirectly. And that latter case has nothing to do with the situation where another person decides that my life should be terminated on extraneous eugenic or social grounds. The fact that all three interventions bring about the same end result, my death, does not mean that they are three species, one 'voluntary', the others 'involuntary', of the same genus 'euthanasia'. In any event, the argument I am proposing puts the emphasis not on a 'happy death' (*eu-thanatos*) but on what might be called an autonomous death, a death that I have as a moral agent, after serious reflection, determined for myself.

The claim that I have a right to determine the manner of my death goes against, of course, traditional religious attitudes to suicide which saw suicide as inspired by cowardice and weakness – a refusal to endure the difficulties and suffering of life – and also, rather ambivalently, by a kind of hubris which led people to usurp the role of God as the arbiter of life and death. The idea that since God gives us life only God can take it away, runs deep in the Judaic and Christian and Islamic traditions, even though it sits rather inconsistently with the status given, by these religious traditions, to the martyr who deliberately offers up her life and dies for God. In the Middle Ages, theologians such as St Thomas Aquinas used a battery of arguments – theological, philosophical and utilitarian – to show that suicide is a sin. Thus Aquinas claims that the deliberate taking of one's life goes against our 'natural' inclination to preserve ourselves; it is a sin against charity since as a matter a charity everyone should cherish or love themselves; it is an offence against the community since every person is a part of the community and what damages each person damages the community; it is an attempt to play God since life is God's gift and God alone has the authority to decide when a person should die.[2] With respect to the last point Aquinas admits that concerning the rest of his life a person must use his free will and make his own autonomous decisions; it is only regarding his death that he must leave the decision to God.[3] Again, Aquinas argues that suicide is not an act of true courage but rather of 'softness of spirit' (*mollities animi*) of a person not able to bear with life's afflictions.

It must be said that much remains unclear in Aquinas's

arguments against suicide. For example, if it is against the natural law (that is, against our 'natural' propensity to preserve our life) to take one's life, does this mean that I have an absolute duty to preserve my life at all costs and that I have a correlative duty to shun occasions where my life is endangered? Contemporary followers of Aquinas certainly do not hold that we have an absolute obligation to preserve life at all costs or that we cannot bring about our death by refusing medical treatment in certain circumstances. Again, if only God can decide when I should die how do I know what God's decision is? Say if I am afflicted with some illness which if left untreated will result in my dying? Should I see the illness as an indication of God's will for me and forgo any medical treatment in a spirit of fatalism? If I had medical treatment would I be defying God's decision that I should die through that illness by having medical treatment? Would having that treatment be tantamount to 'playing God'? Or does the idea that only God can take my life simply (and vacuously) mean that when I die from 'natural causes' (and not from any deliberate act of my own) this is defined as God 'taking my life'? Certainly it is difficult to see why I cannot control the manner of my dying by my free will if, as Aquinas admits, I must control the rest of my life by my free will.

Quite apart from this, Aquinas and other Christian and Jewish and Muslim theologians simply do not consider the possibility that I might in good conscience choose to 'lay down' my life or deliberately terminate my life out of proper self-love, or love for others or for my country or even out of love and respect for God.

Traditional ideas about suicide still, of course, retain some force: in many societies attempted suicide is still seen as a crime and being an accessory to suicide is equally a criminal offence. However, there has been a developing recognition, over the last thirty or forty years, of what has been called a 'right to die'. Like all such catchy slogans, the 'right to die' slogan can be misleading, but what it means is that a person has the right, as an autonomous moral agent, to determine and control the manner of their death, just as they determine and control the manner of their life. Dying is, in a sense, the most important thing a person does and one should as far as possible be in control of it. I do not exercise my moral autonomy by allowing my life to be dictated by chance and external forces, and neither do I exercise my moral autonomy by fatalistically allowing my death to be dictated by chance and external forces. It is not 'playing God' to seek freely to control the direction of my *life*, and it is not 'playing God' to seek freely to control the mode of my dying. For a Christian, God is not honoured by a person (made in the 'image' of God) abdicating her autonomy and freedom of will and passively submitting herself to 'fate'.

The American Catholic moral theologian, Fr Richard A. McCormick, has recently criticised 'physician-assisted suicide' on the grounds that it is based on what he calls the 'absolutisation of autonomy'. Exaggerated emphasis on personal autonomy, he claims, leads to a rejection of dependence on other people and refusal of their compassion.[4] But there is no reason why personal autonomy must be linked with this kind of isolationist and antisocial individualism. Autonomy does not mean that I cannot take advice from others about my life and death or defer to others' opinions, or entrust myself to their care and compassion. It means, however, that in the last resort it is I, this autonomous agent, who has to make such decisions. I cannot abdicate or de-emphasise my personal autonomy since that would be tantamount to abdicating or de-emphasising my status as a moral agent or person. In fact, to complain of the 'absolutisation of autonomy' is rather like complaining of absolutising personhood. Autonomy is not something one can have too much of. As Ronald Dworkin has put it, from another point of view: 'Making someone die in a way that others approve, but he believes is a horrifying contradiction of his life, is a devastating, odious form of tyranny.'[5]

It is worthwhile reflecting here on the traditional Christian idea of a 'good death'. According to this idea death was seen as the natural completion or culmination of a life, the final chapter in, to use a modish term, a life-narrative, and of course in a religious context as a prelude to some other dimension of living. A 'violent death' was one that cut short, in an untimely way, this process of youth, maturity, old age and death.

If we adopt the analogy of a story or narrative and think of a human life as making sense in the way a narrative does – with, as Aristotle says in the *Poetics*, a beginning, a middle and a culminating end – then death will no longer be seen as something intrinsically irrational or 'tragic'.[6] In fact, an endless life in which death played no part would be meaningless: the narrative or story would have no end or point. A good life is one which is not too short and not too long but just right for the expression of the values of a given life.

The idea of a good death represents, of course, an ideal situation and many actual dying situations fall far short of it. But it is worthwhile keeping it in mind as a kind of paradigm by reference to which we can define good caring. Good caring, we might say, is helping or enabling people to die in a humanly meaningful way as the completion or culmination of their lives. That may not always be a happy process of experience in the usual sense of 'happy' but it ought to be a deeply significant process for the dying person. It should not be thought of as a disaster, or as an irrational and senseless evil to be avoided or postponed at all costs.

As against this view of death, there is the view that emerged in the eighteenth and nineteenth centuries with the idea that the human body is a machine. Disease and illness are malfunctions of the body-machine and death is the final mechanical breakdown. The hospital can be seen as the institutional expression of this mechanistic spirit that pervaded science and medicine from the eighteenth century onwards. The American medical sociologist Elliot Mishler, for example, has claimed that the introduction of the machine model into medicine, the professionalisation of medicine and the coming into being of the hospital, all went hand in hand. As he says, 'a machine model of the body is central to the way the profession of medicine entered the twentieth century.'[7]

Mishler also notes that the Flexner Report (1910) redefined the nature of medicine in terms of technology. 'Medical curricula and practice were shaped around what was easily standardised and defined in technological models. To work appropriately and to claim expertise in the late nineteenth and early twentieth centuries was to work with standardised objects defined in isolation from their social context. The body became a standardised object, and the medical curriculum organised around standardisable skills.'[8] As a result death was transformed from a human and religious phenomenon into 'a problem of bodily function'. Attention was directed to the body and – as with so many aspects of nature – it became a machine susceptible to repair and intervention.[9] From this redefinition of health and illness and death, and from the professionalisation of health carers that it led to, the institution of the hospital as we know it developed.

At all events, whatever its historical and socio-cultural origins, the hospital is now in our society the principal context within which health care is provided, and within which death takes place, just as in our society the school is the principal context within which education is provided.

To return to our theme: if the notion of a good death has any meaning as a death that a person chooses and controls, as far as that is possible, for themselves, and represents the culmination of a life-narrative and not just the running down and breakup of a machine, then the notion of palliative care for the dying assumes a new importance. Such care should ideally be seen as a preparation, or even education, for death in the sense just described. Death, it has been said, 'is often attended by conspiracies of silence, alienation, selective attention and false reassurances' and authentic palliative care should have nothing to do with such 'death denying attitudes'.[10]

In this perspective so-called advance health directives have a central place. These advance directives are of different kinds: *living wills* which are legal instruments specifying how a patient wishes to be treated in some future situation where he or she may be incompetent to give consent or make decisions; *durable power of attorney* which is also a legal instrument giving another designated person the right to make decisions for the patient when the latter is incompetent; *informal or non-legal directives* which provide information for relatives, physicians and health care givers about how the patient wishes to be treated if he or she becomes incompetent. In these directives the patient usually specifies what she regards as an unacceptable disability (for example, to be completely bedridden and totally dependent on others, inability to communicate, loss of control over bladder and bowels and so on), what treatment she would want in such a situation (for example, palliative care only with no nasogastric tubes, no resuscitation if she has a cardiac arrest), what she wants done after death (for example, whether she agrees to a post-mortem and to the donation of her organs).[11] Even though these directives may not have any strictly legal force they do provide valuable information to relatives and health care givers about how the patient wishes to die. Recent surveys have shown that there is a great deal of support from the general public for these directives; thus a Canadian study of 909 people has found that a large proportion of the sample wanted to have some control over their future health care and to express their wishes about the future level of care if they were unable to communicate at that time. In answer to the question, 'If unable to communicate, how important would it be to you to have an advance directive indicating the level of care?', 92.3 per cent said that it would be extremely important. And in answer to the question 'Would you want to have your desired level of care documented?', 88.7 per cent said 'yes'.[12] Again, a recent Australian study of 462 subjects found that 80.5 per cent agreed that they would consider nominating someone, in advance, to make decisions about medical treatment on their behalf.[13]

Such directives, however, are limited to medical treatment in mainly terminal situations and other attempts (as in the Victorian *Medical Treatment (Enduring Power of Attorney) Act 1990*) have been made to enlarge their scope to give people an opportunity to reflect more generally upon how they wish to die. An interesting example of this is the directive sponsored by the Center for Health, Law and Ethics at the University of New Mexico in the United States. The first part of the directive, called 'Values History Form', invites people to think about and write down what they think to be important about a number of matters to do with their health: overall attitude to one's health; perception of the role of one's doctor and other health care givers ('Do you trust your doctors?', 'Do you think your doctors should make the final decision concerning any treatment you might need?'); one's thoughts about independence and control ('How important is independence and self-sufficiency in your life?'); one's personal relationships ('What, if any, unfinished business from the past are you concerned about [for example, personal and family relationships, business and legal matters])?'; one's overall attitude to life ('Are you happy to be alive?', 'What do you fear most?'); one's attitudes toward illness, dying and death ('What will be important to you when you are dying [for example, physical comfort, no pain, family members present?]?' 'Where would you prefer to die?'); one's religious background and beliefs ('How do your religious beliefs affect your attitude toward serious or terminal illness?'); one's living environment; one's attitude concerning finances; one's wishes concerning one's funeral. Two final questions ask: 'How would you like your obituary to read?' and 'How would you write a brief eulogy about yourself to be read at your funeral?'[14] Those using the directives are urged to discuss their answers with their families (parents, grandparents, aunts and uncles) and friends. The whole idea behind the directives is that people should reflect on these issues while they are competent and in good health, not when they are in hospital. The directives will then provide a general profile of the patient's 'values history' which will later, if she is then incompetent, help relatives and health care givers to provide the kind of treatment, and eventually the mode of dying - the 'good death' - she desires.

In general, it has been said, these kinds of directives acknowledge 'the fundamental moral importance of competent patients' self-determination interest in deciding about their own health care according to their own values and conception of a good life'. The same observer goes on to say: 'The importance this interest is accorded both in law and medical practice can be seen in the deferral to the competent patient's wishes even when the patient's health or life is sacrificed by doing so, such as in the acceptance of Jehovah's Witness' refusal of life-saving blood transfusions.'[15]

I have been attempting to show how a good death is one over which a person has some degree of control so that it is, to the greatest degree feasible in the circumstances, an expression of that person's life values and of their conception of the good life. A good death is then an autonomous death - a death I choose and determine for myself - and from this point of view it is something that a liberal society should favour and foster in the ways I have described.

NOTES

1. I have elaborated these ideas in a recent book, *Bioethics in a Liberal Society*, Cambridge University Press, Melbourne, 1993.

2. *Summa Theologiae*, 2a, 2ae, 64,5.

3. See *Summa Theologiae*, 2a, 2ae, 64, 5 ad 3.

4. Richard A. McCormick, 'Physician assisted suicide: flight from compassion', *Christian Century*, 108, (1991) 1132.

5. Ronald Dworkin, *Life's Dominion; An Argument About Abortion, Euthanasia and Individual Freedom*, Knopf, New York, 1993, p. 46.

6. See the excellent essay by Brian Scarlett, 'Fastened to a dying animal', *Res Publica*, University of Melbourne, Centre for Philosophy and Public Issues, vol. 2, no. 1, 1993, p. 4.

7. Elliot G. Mishler et al. (eds) *Social Contexts of Health, Illness and Patient Care*, Cambridge University Press, Cambridge, 1981, p. 232.

8. Mishler, p. 232.

9. Mishler, p. 239.

10. See Michael Ashby and Brian Stoffell, 'Therapeutic ratio and defined phases: proposal of ethical framework for palliative care', *British Medical Journal*, 1 June 1991, pp. 1322–24.

11. These details are taken from William Molloy, Virginia Mepham, Roger Clarnette, *Let Me Decide*, Penguin Books, Ringwood, 1993. This is a simple but excellent survey of health care directives and their legal status in Australia.

12. David Molloy, Gordon Guyatt, Efrem Alemayehu, William McIlroy, 'Treatment preferences, attitudes towards advance directives and concerns about health care', *Humane Medicine*, Canada, vol. 7, no. 4, n1991, p. 287.

13. Michael Ashby and Melanie Wakefield, 'Attitudes to some aspects of death and dying, living wills and substituted health care decision-making in South Australia', Public opinion survey for a parliamentary select committee, Government of South Australia, Adelaide, 1993.

14. 'Values History Form', Center for Health, Law and Ethics, School of Law, The University of New Mexico, Albuquerque, NM, USA.

15. Dan W. Brock, 'A proposal for the use of advance directives in the treatment of incompetent mentally ill persons', *Bioethics*, vol. 7, no. 2/3,

1993, p. 256. On the use of advance directives in living organ donation see I. Kleinman and F. H. Lowy, 'Ethical considerations in living donation and a new approach: An advance-directive organ registry', *Bioethics News*, 12 April 1993, pp. 16–22.

The Cacothanasia
of Uncle Albert

My Uncle Albert was a good bloke. He was the sort of man for whom the word avuncular might well have been invented. He was ebullient, funny and kind. He was not an educated or, as far as I was aware, a thoughtful chap. He had grown up in tough times with limited opportunities and he had made the most of them.

Uncle Albert used to let me drive his truck well before I was old enough to hold a driver's licence. Indeed, I used to go out rabbiting in his truck on my own. He had great confidence in other people's abilities to do the right thing and make the right choices.

You know how there are some Aunties and Uncles who, when you see them coming up the drive in their car, make you genuinely happy? Albert was one of those sorts of people. He was a simple, self-reliant, proud man.

Terry Lane was born in Adelaide in 1939. He trained for the Churches of Christ ministry in Melbourne and was a clergyman from 1962 to 1972. He joined the ABC in 1971 as a producer in the Religion Department and then moved into general radio broadcasting. From 1982 to 1983 he presented a daily radio program heard in Melbourne, Sydney, Hobart and Newcastle and on the regional network and Radio Australia. He writes a regular column for the *Sunday Age* in Melbourne, and is the author of six books, including a personal statement on religion and ethics called *God: the interview*, published in 1993.

Albert had a long and healthy life, until in his eighties the cells in his bowel tissue went haywire. He had cancer.

Needless to say the doctors did what they always do. They operated. They removed what they could and fitted Uncle Albert up with a colostomy. He was appalled. It was so undignified to be getting around with a bag of excrement hanging off his body. My guess is that he was the sort of man who was actually embarrassed by all bodily functions, including sex. I never heard him utter a coarse word or tell a dirty joke in the forty-odd years that I knew him. He belonged to that generation and that class of person – the genteel, upwardly-mobile poor – that was uneasy with its body. So I can imagine that the colostomy was mortifying for him.

Nevertheless, that was not the worst of the matter. My guess is that he would have gone on living with his embarrassment, if that had been a choice that he was in a position to make. But he wasn't. The cancer was not eradicated from his system, but further operations and therapy were pointless, so he was sent home to die.

One day the pain in his guts became so excruciating and the bag so humiliating that he went into the wash-house, loaded his old twelve gauge, which hadn't been used for years, and shot himself in the stomach. Aunty G. heard the gun and rushed out to see what had happened and found him on the floor with a massive abdominal wound, but still alive. The ambulance came and he was rushed to hospital and there they worked overtime and with all the skill that the medical profession could muster and they saved his life!

He lived on for a time after that in misery before finally he died *of natural causes.*

Uncle Albert's action in shooting himself in the stomach was ambiguous in its meaning. If he seriously intended to kill himself why did he not shoot himself in the head? The obvious answer to the question is that he wanted to kill the cancer and the pain, not himself. He wanted to live, but without the agony.

Uncle Albert's death troubles me because of the paucity of his choices. In effect he only had two. He could kill himself with great violence or he could endure to the end, with the medical profession (from the most noble motives) squeezing every pain-filled and useless minute out of his life that they could. He was given no other choice.

After shooting himself no one said to him: 'Mr T., may we offer you an easeful death? May we give you a deep and peaceful sleep in which there will be no pain and embarrassment?' And he could not ask for it, because he would not have known enough to know what to ask for.

What if Uncle Albert could have simply gone to his pharmacist and asked for the *Black Pill?* The suicide capsule. The ultimate soporific.

J., who occasionally works near me, watched his wife die a long and painful death, also from cancer. He is angry that she had to endure this final agony. He doesn't want it to happen to him. And he is also angry that the knowledge and the substances which every doctor or pharmacist has at her fingertips is denied to him simply because he is not a member of the fraternity of the medical guild. Why should this knowledge be restricted to men and women with white coats and stethoscopes? He thinks that this is the very worst type of paternalism. How dare they presume to withhold from him the knowledge of the easeful death and keep it to themselves as a black and grim privilege to which lesser mortals may not be admitted. Should J. also be attacked by cancer he wants to be able to decide the time and place of his death. It is his business and no one else's.

I agreed with him. He is absolutely right. So I said: 'J., you are quite right. The knowledge and the chemistry of suicide should be available to everyone. It is outrageous that we should be given only two choices, violent suicide or endurance to the end. We should be able to walk into the chemist shop and say, "I'll have the *Black Pill*, please. No need for a bag, thank you. And that will be all ... "'

J. was appalled. How could I suggest such a thing? What he meant was that the *Black Pill* should be there for *him* when he needs it, but, heaven forfend, not for everyone! Men, women and children suffering from no more than temporary depression would be killing themselves on a whim. No, no. We can't have that.

'So,' I asked him, 'who decides – and by what criteria – who is entitled to get the *Black Pill?*'

J. had no problem with answering that question. It should be available to *him*, because he is intelligent and wise and 'getting on in years'. And how, I asked him, does that differ from the paternalism of the medical profession? Well, it just does!

I imagine that J. would have no problem with making the pill available to Uncle Albert. But, in general, the idea of human moral autonomy terrifies him. He is not alone in that deep-seated aversion to the idea that people should be left alone to make the decisions and choices which they believe will best suit them in the circumstances. J. will not let go of the seductive notion of moral totalitarianism or paternalism. He doesn't trust other people – that's what it boils down to.

We have a distrust of the good sense of our fellow humans that makes us think that they need to be controlled or they will get out of hand doing mischief to themselves and to others. There is no evidence that this is the case, of course – but we believe it fervently, in the absence of any proof from experience that it will in fact be so.

When 6 o'clock closing was abolished there were dire predictions of the imminent collapse of the nation into the gutter of universal drunkenness. It didn't happen. When the divorce laws were changed to make divorce easier the jeremiahs prophesied the end of marriage itself. It didn't come to pass. When censorship laws were changed there was a fear that there would be a sex-crime wave. It simply didn't happen.

Prohibitionists argue that the decriminalisation of drugs would lead to a self-destructive orgy of drug abuse and subsequent addiction that would ruin the nation. Of course sensible people know that it won't happen. Generally speaking humans beings behave prudently because you live longer that way! Humans can be trusted to regulate their own behaviour in their own best interests. In spite of what the pessimists might argue there is no case of a nation going berserk as a consequence of an excess of personal liberty. On the contrary, it is a characteristic of the worst-behaved nations that they are also the societies with the most dedicated and assiduous moral police.

On the other hand, I have never met a decent, well-behaved moderately intelligent middle-class citizen who thought for one moment that *she* needs to be under the watchful eye of the moral guardians. *She* is perfectly capable of monitoring and controlling her own behaviour. But she is much concerned about what her less moral neighbour or her *weaker brother* might get up to if given too much moral leeway.

My friend J. thinks like that. He is adamant that we could trust him with the *Black Pill* – but just off-hand he can't think of anyone else who could be trusted with it.

One of the arguments advanced in support of the censor's ban on Derek Humphry's *Final Exit*[1] was that the book would fall into the wrong hands and teenagers would be dying like flies by their own hands because they would now possess the magical knowledge of the painless death. 'In other words,' I said to J., 'you are telling me that it is a good idea to make suicide as violent, painful and messy as possible because we need that deterrent to prevent an epidemic of DIY deaths?' Yes – that is exactly what he does think.

Final Exit has been available in the shops for some time

now. I am not aware of a sudden epidemic of suicide that could be attributed to the book.

In the time that it was banned I offered to make copies of the book for anyone who wanted it. And I meant *anyone*. I would not judge whether or not they were somehow or other more morally entitled to the information in it than any other person. In the end I made twelve copies and sent them out to people who asked for them. It was my small gesture of civil disobedience in the cause of human moral autonomy. I am not aware that anyone to whom I gave the book has yet used the information in it to commit suicide.

If I had had a letter from a person who said: 'I am 18 years old and very depressed and I am thinking of ending my life. Please send the book', I am not certain what I would have done. As it happened all the people who asked for it were obviously adults past middle age. Should I have sent a book to an unhappy teenager? Well, now they can go into a bookshop and buy it anyway, so why not?

Freedom never comes without risks. It is ludicrous to think that we can set some people free from the moral tyranny of the Church and State without running the risk that some individuals will misuse this freedom. So what? That's life. If J. wants the *Black Pill* then he has to accept the uncertainties that are inevitably attendant on the exercise of his own rights as a human being.

We are not yet free of the tentacles of the coercive Church and State. I read recently that the Vatican (in response to events in Bosnia) says that women in danger of rape may use contraceptives, because 'rape is an act of violence, to which the rules applying to an act within marriage cannot apply.' What's more, although the absolute prohibition on abortion remains, some Roman Catholic bishops in England and Wales reckon that it is morally permissible for rape victims to use the 'morning after pill'. I wonder how the stocks of morning after pills are holding up in Sarajevo? Do they get priority in

United Nations relief-supply convoy cargoes?

You see, what is offensive about this casuistry is that it is based on the assumption that the women of Bosnia are not free moral agents with the birth-given right to make the moral choices that best suit themselves in the circumstances in which they find themselves. The bishops are fools. It is hard to find a good word to say about them. They presume to grant a moral boon which is not within their prerogative. They do not own the bodies, intelligence or consciences of the women of Bosnia.

The Roman Catholic Church of Australia has fought a ferocious rearguard action against contraception, abortion, sterilisation and divorce. Popes have even at some times opposed vaccination and anaesthesia as being an affront to the will of God. The Church has lost every one of these battles. Now the issue of suicide is the Church's last stand.

Over the centuries the Church has had a peculiar and contradictory attitude to death. Christians have taken a suspect sadomasochistic delight in the sufferings and deaths of Jesus and the martyrs while at the same time holding to this notion that somehow suicide is an offence to the Almighty. In its earliest anarchistic, pacifist days the Church was possibly consistent in its attitude to the sanctity of life, but from the time of Constantine onwards the Roman Catholic Church has never hesitated to encourage and bless unnatural and untimely death on a massive scale through war, crusades and the persecution of dissidents. Indeed the Church has, by and large, been in love with death. It is one of the most murderous institutions the world has ever seen, committing and excusing appalling atrocities in the name of God. Yet it cavils at contraception, abortion and suicide. It is hard to envisage a grander, more repulsive hypocrisy than this and it is hard to explain.

But hard to explain or not, it infects our thinking. We are reluctant to let go of the idea that we are Fallen and sinful creatures who need to be morally managed and controlled by guardians of conscience who claim to be appointed to the job by God Herself. It is a tribute to the thoroughness with which the Church has done its job that we don't laugh out loud at the preposterous presumption built into this assertion of moral totalitarianism.

It may seem that I am laying unduly heavy blame on the Roman Catholic Church for our present cowardly and befuddled thinking on suicide, but I do so because I believe that it is only the intimidation of the Church that keeps politicians in a moral funk. They know what they ought to do, but they are terrified of stirring up the bishops and perhaps running the risk of losing a Catholic vote or two. The Victorian legislature went to water on the matter of 'living wills' when the Catholic Archbishop of Melbourne shook his crook. The premier at the time even gave the Bishop an assurance that nothing would be enacted that would be offensive to Catholics. It is possible that most intelligent politicians will happily concede in private that what a person chooses to do about the time and manner of her death is entirely her own business, but they will not say that in public for the simple and single reason that it will cause a noisy response from the Church. So, votes being more important than the intellectual or moral well-being of the community, they keep silent.

However, the good news is that bit by bit we are breaking free of the malign moral tyranny of the Church. No matter how much the bishops may protest there is no doubt that every day more and more people are questioning the morality or the wisdom of prolonging life beyond the point where it loses meaning.

The anti-Nazi martyr, Dietrich Bonhoeffer, in his *Ethics*, devotes a chapter to suicide. He writes with sympathy of the suicide.

Suicide is a man's attempt to give a final human meaning to a life which has become humanly meaningless. The involuntary sense of horror which seizes us when we are faced with the fact of a suicide is not to be attributed to the iniquity of such a deed but to the terrible loneliness and freedom in which this deed is performed, a deed in which the positive attitude to life is reflected only in the destruction of life.[2]

I could wish that he had left it there, but he could not resist the temptation of presuming to know what God is thinking. 'God has reserved to Himself the right to determine the end of life, because He alone knows the goal to which it is His will to lead.'[3] But that, as we know, was not the last word on the divine prerogative over life. Bonhoeffer took part in the plot to assassinate Hitler. He did not trust his God to 'determine the end of life' for the Führer. He took matters into his own hands. In other words, he took proper human responsibility in those circumstances, rather than passively leaving it to the Almighty to determine the outcome of events and life itself. We venerate the memory of Bonhoeffer precisely because he took matters into his own hands, even though in doing so he committed himself to two possible outcomes. Either the plot would succeed, in which case Bonhoeffer would be a murderer – or it would fail, in which case Bonhoeffer was committing suicide. He didn't leave much scope for the action of God in his deeds.

We put such a lot of effort and ingenuity into postponing death that suicide seems so bizarre and unnatural that we readily succumb to the false arguments in favour of the maintenance of the 'Everlasting's canon 'gainst self-slaughter'. Some people assume that other people with self-destructive inclinations need to be protected from themselves. They have difficulty accepting that in some circumstances suicide is the sensible choice to make. As Bonhoeffer says, it is the act of 'terrible loneliness and freedom'[4] that shows how seriously the person values life.

My friend J. has an unreasonable fear that if the *Black Pill* were on sale at the local chemist shop there would be a rash of suicides. But common sense tells us that this would not be so. The will to live is so powerful that we know intuitively that life needs to be really grim and meaningless before it becomes less attractive than death.

But this is the easy stuff. Suicide, committed by a person in full possession of her faculties, is not a big deal for any sensible person. The big moral dilemmas involve the question of helping other people to commit suicide. Then a third party – perhaps a doctor – must get involved in the act. Or, as is often the case, the courts will be asked to pass judgment on a man or a woman who has helped a spouse to die. Here we enter a gloomy twilight world of the morally ambiguous where it is simply not possible to write laws that will cover all possible situations.

Consider my poor Uncle Albert. The doctor could have prescribed some narcotic for him and sent him away to work out for himself how he would use it. We might judge the doctor in those circumstances to be doing no more than increasing the choices available to a dying man. But what if the dying man wants more – a lethal injection there and then? How will we judge the doctor then? And what if the wife or child of the dying man gets involved as an agent? How shall we judge? And what if the man has expressed a deep desire for release from suffering and then immediately goes into a coma and is no longer competent to give the final assent? Should the suicide assistants proceed? And every minute that they hesitate to take the fatal action makes them more guilty of killing a person who is not in a position to give consent, even though his wishes have been expressed clearly enough in the recent past.

From time to time old men kill their demented wives or old women help their beloved husbands to die with some dignity. Usually they are dealt with kindly by the courts. We turn a tearful eye from the spectacle. Punishment is unthinkable.

At this point, it seems to me, we are up against the barrier of the limits of law. It is simply not possible to write laws covering these cases. The written statute on the subject of killing has to be absolute, stern and inflexible. At no time and in no circumstances is it permissible for one human being to kill another. That's it. There can be no exceptions in the written law.

But ... Except ... There is a territory on the fringes of human experience where the law ceases to make sense. It is not possible to write a statute so subtle and so prescient that it could foresee every possible eventuality and prescribe and proscribe the proper and improper behaviour in those circumstances. Laws can only describe the 'normal' – but beyond the limits of the normal there are the situations which are unique. How we decide and judge and act in those circumstances is of necessity *ad hoc.*

I cannot envisage any law that will cover all circumstances. Some relatives and doctors will consider it their moral duty to prolong life – others will take it as their melancholy moral duty to help to die. In the end we cannot say with certainty who is right and who is wrong. In these circumstances the stern and inflexible objectivity of the law must make way for the uncertainties inherent in compassion and empathy. 'Judge not, and you will not be judged; condemn not and you will not be condemned; forgive and you will be forgiven ... '

I realise that many people are terrified of this sort of moral circumstantialism. They fear that in the absence of laws which are universal and unaffected by circumstances we will sink into a state of destructive moral anarchy. Well, I don't believe that. There are times when lying or stealing is justified – any imaginative person can easily think up situations in which you would be morally justified in lying or stealing. And most such people could also think of situations in which even killing might be justified. But it is not possible to write laws that say: 'Thou shalt not lie, except in the following circumstances.'

We are far too reverential and uncritical in our attitudes to the written statute and so tend to deprive people of the necessity of acting as moral beings. There are times when it is necessary to 'do what is best in the circumstances', never mind what the law might say. The State may then choose to examine the situation and the motives of the actors in the moral drama and to judge with mercy if the circumstances suggest that is appropriate. As unsatisfactory as this may seem it is the best that we can hope for in a less than perfect world.

It will mean that sometimes a husband, like Derek Humphry, may help a wife to commit suicide. Sometimes a wife may help her husband die because she can no longer bear to watch the suffering of the one she loves and who is begging for release from pain and indignity. It is simply inconceivable that we should write rules to cover these events. But we should nevertheless *expect* them. We should be mature enough to regard them as sad but inevitable little dramas in the grand play of human existence.

Creative thinkers are beavering away at the edges of this moral dilemma, devising living wills and writing legislation that would give the doctors the right in certain circumstances to assist a suicide. But in the end the law will not give us the comfort of certainty that we crave. We must learn to come to terms with moral uncertainty and ambiguity. And in the end those who help another person take her life can never know for certain that they have done the good rather than the evil deed.

That they have done a serious deed must never be doubted. If the day came when we regarded the taking of a human life, no matter how diminished, as a thing of no consequence then we would indeed be in moral trouble. But to regard an act with great gravity does not mean that it must be automatically condemned as wicked. Sometimes the difference between wickedness and virtue can only be discerned in the motives of the agents and the circumstances in which they act and in the consequences of their deeds.

One day I was interviewing a doctor on my wireless program. He was telling me how to prolong my life. I should eat less meat and more high-fibre vegetables. I should definitely not smoke, nor should I go out in the noonday sun without a hat and a neck-to-ankle burnous to protect me from the ultraviolet rays. I should exercise every day and avoid all foods that tend to raise the cholesterol level. Indeed, to really squeeze the last minute out of life I would be well-advised to emulate the lifestyle of Seventh Day Adventists, he said.

Well, I said, if I do all that you advise I will never get cancer, heart disease or a stroke. So how will I die? What is the best – the 'natural' – way to shuffle off this mortal coil?

Another doctor who heard the program wrote to me as follows. 'The natural, and best, death is to snuff it at 87 from terminal *coitus interruptus* brought on by being shot by a jealous husband.'

'Tis a consummation devoutly to be wish'd.

NOTES

1. Derek Humphry, *Final Exit*, Penguin, Ringwood, 1992.
2. Dietrich Bonhoeffer, *Ethics*, Collins, London, 1964 [first published in Germany under the title *Ethik* by Chr. Kaiser Verlag, 1949] p. 167.
3. Bonhoeffer, p. 168.
4. Bonhoeffer, p. 168.

Pieter Admiraal

Listening and Helping to Die: the Dutch Way

I have been a doctor for nearly forty years and am now Senior Anaesthetist at the Reinier de Graaf Gasthuis, a large 800-bed general hospital in the Dutch city of Delft. My role is not only that of a traditional anaesthetist; since the late 1960s, I have also specialised in pallia-tive care, that is, in pain and symptom control for the incura-bly ill and dying and have been a member of the hospital's Ter-minal Care Team since it was officially set up in 1973.

As a member of that team, I also practise active voluntary euthanasia – openly and unas-hamedly. I practise it openly because I am fortunate to live in a country that allows doctors to do so. And I practise it unasha-medly because I regard it as sometimes morally right, as not only *compatible* with the prop-erly understood duties and

Pieter Admiraal is a Senior Anaesthetist at a large general hospital in the Dutch city of Delft. He first performed active voluntary euthanasia some twenty years ago, in what was then a Roman Catholic hospital.

In 1992, Pieter Admiraal was presented with the International Humanist Award in recognition of his advocacy of the humanist value of self-determination in the field of voluntary euthanasia where his pioneering work has positively influenced the attitude of the medical profession and the general public in the Netherlands and other countries.

responsibilities of a doctor, but as an act sometimes *required* by them. To fail to practise voluntary euthanasia under some circumstances is to fail the patient.

Here I want to recount the cases of two patients who requested active help in dying – Carla and Esther. Carla suffered from terminal cancer; Esther from the incurable and progressively debilitating disease multiple sclerosis.[1]

Carla[2] was 47 years old. She was married to Henk, and the couple had four teenage children. Late in 1988, Carla noticed a painful swelling in her lower abdomen and went to her family doctor. He referred her to a gynaecologist at the Delft hospital, where I practise.

A subsequent operation revealed that the pain had been caused by a large malignant tumour on one of Carla's ovaries. By the time the operation was performed, the tumour had already grown so large that it could not be totally removed.

Carla underwent chemotherapy and by June her condition had greatly improved. She felt relatively well until March 1990, when it was found that the tumour had regrown. Chemotherapy was tried once more, but this time it was in vain.

By the middle of the year, Carla's pain had increased to such an extent that her family doctor had to prescribe opioids (morphine-like drugs). Her condition deteriorated quickly and it was not long before Carla had to be readmitted to our hospital. This is when I saw her for the first time in my role as palliative care specialist.

I told Carla that I would almost certainly be able to relieve her pain. This proved correct. A needle placed under her skin delivered a continuous infusion of morphine, and after two days Carla's pain was well controlled. She was, of course, greatly relieved. But, like many patients in her situation, she was afraid that the pain would steadily get worse and that it would, in the end, not be possible to control it.

I visited Carla at least once a day. During one of those visits, she raised the question of euthanasia: would she be helped to die when the stage had been reached where she found her condition unbearable? Her husband, Henk, was visibly upset by his wife's request. Whilst he understood that there was ultimately nothing more that could be done to save his wife's life, he had not as yet realised that he would lose her so soon. I explained to Carla that doctors at this hospital were always willing to listen, and that we did not regard the question of voluntary euthanasia as a taboo subject. But, I also pointed out to her, the final decision could not be made unilaterally by a patient or her doctor. It had to be agreed to by a team consisting of two doctors, a nurse, and one of the hospital's spiritual caregivers – the Roman Catholic chaplain, the Protestant chaplain, or the Humanist counsellor.

On the next day, Carla was already discussing the question of euthanasia with the hospital's Roman Catholic chaplain, who was sympathetic to her request.

From then on, her condition deteriorated quickly. She was vomiting constantly. For psychological reasons, Carla was still taking fluids by mouth, even though this would almost immediately lead to vomiting. To avoid this incessant vomiting, it became necessary to put a tube through her nose into her stomach. This way, we could constantly evacuate her stomach. To prevent thirst, Carla received an infusion of a saline solution. When the question arose whether she should also be fed intravenously, Carla decided against this, not wanting to prolong her life unnecessarily.

Carla lost a lot of weight and became extremely weak, unable even to move around in her bed. This made it very difficult for the nurses to prevent bedsores. While Carla lost weight, the tumour continued to grow and was soon obstructing the blood flow in her legs, causing them to swell painfully.

Right from the time of her admission to the hospital, Carla had had a room of her own. This meant that her family could visit her freely, and it became customary for Henk and one of the children to sleep in the same room. She was also frequently visited by her family doctor and his wife.

Throughout her illness, Carla remained completely alert. She was a courageous woman. Not only did she bear her own physical deterioration bravely, she also provided emotional support for her family. She was sustained by a strong Catholic faith, and was convinced that she would live on in heaven.

When the time of her death seemed near, the Catholic chaplain administered the Last Sacraments. Soon after, Carla requested us – not unexpectedly – to end her suffering. 'God could not have wanted this,' she said. By this time, her husband had also come to accept her wish to die. He had realised that it would be selfish of him not to let his wife go.

A family meeting was called. The eldest son still clung to the hope that his mother might get better and found it difficult to accept her decision. However, after Carla had talked to him privately, he, too, agreed with her decision.

Similarly the nurses, who had cared for Carla on a daily basis: they knew her circumstances well and respected Carla's wish to die. Then the gynaecologist, the Roman Catholic chaplain and I discussed the case, and were all of the opinion that the patient's wish should be respected.

In situations such as these, we always hesitate. A patient's request for euthanasia may, after all, be a cry for help – prompted perhaps by shortcomings in the delivery of palliative care. This was not true in Carla's case. She had received the best of care, and there was nothing more that could be done to alleviate her suffering.

Carla was visited once more by the family doctor and his wife. They had come to say farewell. Then Carla and I met with the family. It was arranged that euthanasia would be performed on the following day, and Carla signed the relevant consent form.

When the day had come, Carla once again confirmed her

wish to die. Her husband, Henk, two of Carla's sisters, her parish priest, and two of the children were by her side when I administered the drugs which would give her the benign death she desired. Carla fell asleep with a smile on her face. She died eight minutes later, on 6 August 1990.

There are those who will be shocked by the case of Carla. They will be shocked because I took deliberate steps to end Carla's life. By injecting a lethal drug, they will say, I killed Carla – and killing a patient is always morally wrong. The fact that Carla was terminally ill, was suffering greatly, and desperately wanted to die, those critics might say, does not make the action morally right.

I take a contrary view: I believe it was morally proper to help Carla die in the way we did. We could have declined, of course, as some doctors do, firmly closing our ears to the patient's request for active help in dying, and Carla would have died, in a day or two, from 'natural causes'. Whilst this approach is the traditional one, I believe it has little to recommend itself from the medical or moral point of view.

As doctors we have two primary duties: to ensure the well-being of our patients, and to respect their autonomy. The first duty entails that we should seek to restore patients to health and, if we can't, that we should try to reduce their suffering. The second duty entails that we listen closely to, and respect, the wishes of our patients. Suffering, loss of control, and physical decline are subjective experiences, and nobody but the patient herself is in a position to decide when enough is enough. It would be quite improper for doctors or other health care professionals to impose their values and their understanding of pain or suffering on the patient.

Even societies which do not allow active voluntary euthanasia do grant patients the freedom to refuse medical treatment. They grant competent people the right to bring their lives to an end by requesting doctors to stop treatment, and doctors have a recognised legal duty to abide by the competent and fully informed patient's request. This is one way of ending life – sometimes referred to as 'passive voluntary euthanasia'. Here the doctor does not administer a lethal drug, but discontinues treatment and the patient will then die of so-called natural causes. Whilst people sometimes refer to these non-treatment decisions as 'passive euthanasia', I believe the term 'euthanasia' is quite misplaced here. 'Euthanasia' means 'a good death', or 'bringing about a good death'. Letting a patient die of her disease may be anything but a good death. The patient may die slowly and painfully, and in what she regards as an undignified manner.

The traditional view is that these 'passive' life-shortening acts are somehow morally better than the 'active' kind: that a doctor who respects a patient's desire to die by discontinuing life-support acts as a good doctor should; a doctor who 'actively' helps a patient like Carla to die, on the other hand, acts morally wrongly. Why?

There is now a large body of philosophical and theological literature on the moral distinction between so-called active and passive voluntary euthanasia. After having studied this sometimes rather convoluted debate, I have reached the conclusion that there is, in the end, no morally relevant difference between these two forms of euthanasia. In both cases, the doctor acts out of respect for the autonomy of the patient. In both cases life is shortened. In both cases, the doctor has performed an act which has led to the patient's death; and in both cases, the doctor must take responsibility for that action – regardless of whether this involves, say, turning off a respirator (supposedly an act of passive euthanasia), or the administration of a lethal injection. As Helga Kuhse has put it:

Stripped of all other differences, what remains is ... a difference that has no moral significance. In active euthanasia, the doctor initiates a course of events that will lead to the patient's death. In letting die [or passive euthanasia], the agent stands back and lets nature take her sometimes cruel course. Is letting die morally better than helping to die, or active euthanasia? I think not. Very often it is much worse.[3]

I agree. Very often passive euthanasia is morally worse than active euthanasia. It is morally worse in all those cases where we inflict on the patient a way of dying that he or she does not want, and finds unacceptable and undignified. In these cases we fail to respect the patient's autonomy; we fail to take seriously that patient's own evaluation of suffering and pain. In short, we fail to respect the patient as a self-determining person.

Fortunately, in most cases it is possible to make dying easier. Sometimes this may require the administration of opioids and sedatives in such high doses that life will be directly shortened by the medication. If this is the case, then it is even more difficult to detect any difference between this practice and active euthanasia: the patient's death is caused by the administration of a drug – just as it is in the case of active euthanasia.

I know what some people will say here. They will say that the doctor merely intended to relieve the patient's pain and that he or she did not intend to kill the patient. But to say this is once again an attempt to evade moral responsibility. Surely, doctors must be held responsible for the deaths they deliberately cause – irrespective of what they say their intentions are. Moreover, this traditional response also fails to take account of the reality of medical practice, where it is often very difficult to distinguish between the different intentions and motivations that lead doctors and patients to adopt one course of action rather than another.

Not many patients will, in the end, ask for active voluntary euthanasia.[4] In the majority of cases, it is possible to ease the dying process and to allow patients to die with dignity.

As I mentioned before, in our hospital in Delft a Terminal Care Team was officially set up in 1973. This team functions in accordance with widely accepted principles of palliative care. We always treat patients as persons, not as the carriers of symptoms or diseases. We recognise the importance of communication, and provide dying patients with an opportunity to discuss their fears of dying; we tell them about the kind of terminal care that can be offered, and we assure them that we will neither abandon them, nor force medical treatment on them that they do not want.

It is sometimes suggested that one of the reasons why voluntary euthanasia has gained a foothold in the Netherlands is that palliative care is not very advanced in our country. This criticism is unjustified. While we have only two hospices, which cater specifically for those who are dying, we have integrated palliative care into the delivery of health care as a whole. Hospices in England, for example, cater for 25 per cent of dying patients. In our country, patients can receive excellent terminal care in either hospitals, (40 per cent), nursing homes (10 per cent), or in their own homes, (50 per cent).

Another misleading claim is that modern methods of pain control will obviate the need for active voluntary euthanasia: that patients will not ask for euthanasia if their pain is adequately controlled. This is an argument frequently voiced by opponents of voluntary euthanasia – both in the Netherlands and in other parts of the world.

Two comments need to be made on this. Firstly, it is true, great advances have been made regarding pain control. Nonetheless, it remains a sad medical fact that in some 5 per cent of cases pain cannot be controlled even with the most advanced techniques, and in some cases it can be controlled only through the continuous intravenous infusion of opioids and other drugs that will render the patient unconscious.

Secondly, pain is very seldom the sole reason why patients request euthanasia. A recent nationwide study has shown that patients ask for active euthanasia because of loss of strength and fatigue, loss of human dignity, and complete dependence. In only 5 per cent of all cases was pain the sole reason for the request.[5]

Even the best of palliative care cannot alleviate all suffering, cannot always make it bearable. Speaking about suffering in the wider sense, Dame Cicely Saunders, the founder of the modern palliative care movement and an opponent of active voluntary euthanasia, agrees: 'Sometimes unrealistic fears can be explained and eased, but a good deal of suffering has to be lived through. The very pain itself may lead to a resolution or a new vision, as came to Job.'[6] These words reflect Dame Cicely's Christian approach to life, death and suffering. I respect that view, but as a doctor I must also respect the views of patients who take a radically different approach.

Of course, we always hesitate if a patient asks for euthanasia. After all, a request for active euthasnasia does not, as such, legitimate its implementation. As a first step, we will always investigate whether the patient has received adequate care and whether there is something else that can be done. But when all is said and done, we must face the fact that it is not possible to relieve all suffering. We cannot protect patients against total physical and psychological disintegration; we cannot protect some of our patients against complete loss of human dignity. We have learnt not to ignore those facts, but have come to accept that some of our patients, in spite of the best possible medical, nursing and spiritual care, will request euthanasia.

Palliative care is essential. It must always be an integral part of good medical care and voluntary euthanasia can never replace it. At our hospital and in our country we do, however, acknowledge the fact that good terminal care must incorporate at least the possibility of voluntary euthanasia. Even if a patient will never request it, the knowledge alone that we are willing to listen to requests for help in dying will alleviate much anxiety and fear, and will give many of those who are nearing the end of their lives peace of mind. And in those instances where we do perform active voluntary euthanasia, we do not regard it as separate from the delivery of terminal care, but rather as the last dignified act of terminal care.

Should active voluntary euthanasia be restricted to those who are terminally ill, that is, to those who are suffering from a disease such as cancer, likely to lead to death in a few days' time?

The notion of 'terminal illness' is slippery. In one sense of the term, we are all terminally ill. As human beings we are mortal and, one day, will have to die. Also, many life-threatening medical conditions will become 'terminal' only once we decide not to treat them. Patients who experience respiratory failure are in mortal danger, but to the extent that we are able to keep them alive with the help of a machine – for months or years perhaps – they are not terminally ill. These patients become 'terminally ill' only once the decision has been made to discontinue life-support.

This means that the notion of terminal illness cannot be employed, in a straightforward way, to justify medical end-of-life decisions. Rather, it becomes necessary to reflect on the values on which medical end-of-life decisions ought to be based. As I said before, I take it that doctors should, on the one hand, seek to maximise the patient's welfare; but that they must, on the other, respect the patient's autonomy. To respect the patient's autonomy presupposes that the patient's own evaluation of her medical situation ought to be the determinative one. The doctor might think that life with a certain condition is, or ought to be, bearable; but to the extent that the properly counselled and supported patient takes a different view, it is the patient's view which must ultimately be the determinative one.

The case of Esther will illustrate the point.

In June, 1983 I was asked to see **Esther**, a young patient in a denominational nursing home, who was asking for active euthanasia. Esther was suffering from multiple sclerosis, a disease of the nervous system. This disease is usually progressive and, in due course, will often completely paralyse the patient.

When I met Esther, she was sitting in an electric wheelchair, unable to walk or move on her own. She could only use her left hand to drive the wheelchair, with the assistance of a nurse. Her breathing was laboured, and she could only speak in short sentences, and with great effort. After an hour, she was completely exhausted.

She told me that she had experienced the first neurological symptoms in 1976. In 1981 she had been admitted to the nursing home, and by the beginning of 1983 she was almost completely paralysed. She had one young daughter and was divorced.

Esther had carefully informed herself about the disease and had reached the conclusion that she would wish to die once she had become completely paralysed and was totally dependent on the care of others. She knew that she would, at some stage, no longer be able to eat by herself; she would not even be able to swallow the food that somebody else had placed in her mouth. If she was not to starve to death, she would need to be fed by way of a tube leading directly into her stomach. But, Esther had decided, she would never accept tube feeding.

In 1982, Esther executed a so-called 'living will', indicating that she did not wish to be kept alive if she were no longer able to communicate her wishes. She also wrote farewell letters to her daughter, members of her family and her friends. Soon after, she had discussed with the director of the nursing home her desire to die. But, Esther said, she was told that there was nothing that could be done for her, 'for religious reasons'.

Unable to obtain help, Esther began to think about suicide; she contemplated the idea of hurling herself and her wheelchair down the stairs, but then dismissed the idea because she was not sure that it would have the desired result. Finally, a friend of hers had got in touch with me.

I visited Esther in the nursing home. When I asked her why she wanted to die, she answered:

Would you like to live under these circumstances? I can't do anything. I am completely dependent on others. I have no future, no outlook, and I'm very afraid that I will suffocate because of the aspiration of food. I've even got to call somebody if there's a fly on my face. This is senseless and cruel, and I want to die as soon as possible.

I asked her about her daughter. Would she not wish to live for the sake of her child. 'My child,' she answered, 'I've not held her in my arms for years; she never had a real mother who could walk with her in the park, feeding ducks and doing similar things ... I can't even buy a present for her; I can't educate her ... I have written a farewell letter to her, which she can read after my death, explaining why I want to die.'

Her doctor confirmed that Esther had difficulties swallowing and that there was a real danger that food would be lodged in her windpipe. This could happen at any time. The result could be pneumonia, but it might also be suffocation. It had been suggested that a feeding tube be put in place, but Esther had refused.

I asked Esther whether she was willing to stop eating, to prove her desire to die was sincere. She indicated that she was willing to do this, but then said that she thought it was very cruel of me to force her to do this. 'Why should I have to suffer first, before you help me die?'

I apologised and explained that it was necessary for me to

be absolutely certain that her wish to die was sincere.

When Esther had left the room, staff of the nursing home confirmed that she had consistently expressed the desire to die and that there was no doubt that she fully understood her circumstances. But, I was told, it was out of the question that any life-shortening act would be performed on the premises.

Instead, Esther was visited by the staff psychologist. But, as soon as he mentioned green pastures, blue skies and butterflies, Esther asked him to leave her room.

After extensive consultation with Esther, her family and friends, it was decided that she would be admitted to our hospital in Delft. Esther was much relieved and, after admission, told us how happy she was that she now had the assurance that she would be helped to die.

A long meeting took place between Esther's parents, some of her friends, our head nurse, the hospital's Roman Catholic chaplain and myself. We subsequently told Esther how difficult it was for us to reach a decision: on the one hand, we respected her wish to die; on the other we were all hesitating. Since she had entered the hospital, she appeared happy and it seemed incongruous to us that she wished her life to end. We even suggested that she should consider admittance to a local nursing home in Delft, where she could stay until she felt that she did not want to go on.

Esther smiled and said: 'This is not what you have promised me – to go to another nursing home and wait for aspiration. That would only prolong my suffering. I can understand that you are hesitating, but you are not aware of what is going on in my mind.'

We were all very impressed by her honest way of speaking and her absolute self-assurance. Nonetheless, we felt it important to seek further advice and consulted Dr Kuitert, a well-known ethicist and theologian from the University of Amsterdam. He took the view that Esther's desire to die was reasonable under the circumstances, and that we should seriously consider honouring her request.

The members of the health care team, including the Roman Catholic chaplain, thought long and hard about the matter, and during the next four days each of us had long and intimate discussions with Esther. In the end, we unanimously agreed that we should honour her wish and that we would end her life.

Esther's parents and best friends came to say goodbye, and to be with her when she died. Esther told us this was the happiest day in her life since she had become ill; she could hardly wait for me to start the infusion. It was an emotional moment. We all cried. We were sad that the life of this unique person had come to an end; but we were glad that we had released her from a life that she found unbearable.

I was subsequently prosecuted for having performed an unlawful act of voluntary euthanasia – presumably because the patient had not been in the terminal phase of her illness. At the hearing, Dr Kuitert gave evidence to the effect that he believed my action was morally acceptable, justified and humane; and a second witness, the Secretary of the Dutch Medical Association, declared that my handling of the case was an example of good medical care, as accepted by the Association. The prosecution was dropped.

When it was all over, I received a letter from the management of my hospital, which congratulated me on the 'clear and satisfying verdict', and the Roman Catholic chaplain wrote: 'The verdict of the court is so unequivocally and pleasingly positive that I want to congratulate you. It is good that the question of good medical care has been answered in all clearness along this unexpected line.'

The outcome of this court case confirms that it is legally permissable for doctors to practise active voluntary euthanasia not only in situations of terminal illness, but also when a patient who is not terminally ill seeks release from a medical condition that imposes unrelievable and unbearable suffering.

Opponents of active voluntary euthanasia will regard this development as yet another step on the so-called 'slippery slope', which will ultimately lead Dutch society to some terrible disaster, where patients will be killed against their will.

I do not accept that there is a slippery slope. A clear moral and legal boundary can be drawn around the notion of consent. This notion of consent, based on respect for the patient's autonomy, is the centrepiece and backbone of the legal framework governing voluntary euthanasia in the Netherlands. Over the last ten years or so, it has served us well. No patient – no matter how ill – will have his or her life cut short, unless there is an explicit request. Active voluntary euthanasia is but one more way of delivering humane medical care.[7]

The Bishop of Durham, Lord Jenkins, recently said that in his opinion voluntary euthanasia, under agreed conditions and surrounded by safeguards, could be part of proper medical care. In these circumstances, he felt, there was no danger of inserting a wedge to split up the curing and caring vocation of doctors, nor of encouraging doctors or relatives to press for the early removal of difficult patients. He said, 'We are working at the next stage of humanizing our mutual care for one another from conception to death.'[8]

In the Netherlands, there is after all these years no evidence of a slippery slope, or of a disturbed relationship between doctors and patients. On the contrary, the acceptance of active voluntary euthanasia has improved the relationship. Patients know that they can count on their doctors when they need them most: when, because of terminal or incurable illness they are vulnerable, and in danger of being denied the basic human right to say: 'Enough is enough. I want to die with my dignity intact. Please help me.'

NOTES

1. The names in these cases are fictitious, to protect the privacy of those involved.
2. A description of this case has previously been published in Pieter V. Admiraal: 'A Physician's Responsibility to Help a Patient Die', (ed.) Robert I. Misbin, *Euthanasia: The Good of the Patient, the Good of Society*, University Publishing Group, Frederic, Maryland, 1992, pp. 77–78.
3. Helga Kuhse, 'The Case for Active Voluntary Euthanasia', *Law, Medicine and Healthcare*, vol. 14, 1987, pp. 145–48.
4. See P. J. van der Maas et al, 'Euthanasia and other medical decisions concerning the end of life', *The Lancet*, vol. 338, 14 Sept. 1991, pp. 669–74.
5. ibid.
6. C. S. Saunders, 'Spiritual Pain', *Journal of Palliative Care*, vol. 4, 1988, pp. 29–32.
7. In her concluding chapter, Helga Kuhse outlines the Dutch regulations governing the practice of active voluntary euthanasia. There is also another discussion of the so-called 'slippery slope' argument.
8. D. E. Jenkins: 'Why not choose death in the end?', *Care of the Critically Ill*, vol. 7, no. 6, 1991, p. 6.

Helga Kuhse

Accepting Responsibility: Dying in Australia and the Netherlands

Pieter Admiraal's thoughtful essay shows how compassionate doctors might responsibly and sensitively respond to an incurably ill patient's wish to die if they are fortunate enough to be practising in a country like the Netherlands that permits them to do so. Many of the Australian contributions, on the other hand, demonstrate how costly – in terms of physical and emotional pain – it is for a country to deny its citizens the right to die. Our existing laws are the result of a particular religious and cultural tradition, which is an inappropriate basis for public policies in liberal, pluralist societies. The anguish and the denial of personal freedom that follow in the wake of our present policies provide very strong arguments for a re-evaluation of our approach.

Does a person who is incurably ill, who suffers much and wants to die, have a right to bring her life to an end, and is it proper for others to help her in this quest? We know from historians and anthropologists that different cultures and peoples have given radically different answers to this question. Some have condemned suicide and voluntary euthanasia – even in the face of great suffering – as cowardly and wrong, while others have praised a self-chosen death as courageous and as an expression of our ultimate freedom as human beings.

The great pre-Christian philosopher Seneca was among

those who thought it was better to choose one's death than endure a life of misery and suffering right to one's natural end. As he put it:

I will not abandon old age, if old age preserves me intact as regards the better part of myself; but if old age begins to shatter my mind, and to pull its various faculties to pieces, if it leaves me not life, but only the breath of life, I shall rush out of a house that is crumbling and tottering. I shall not avoid illness by seeking death, as long as the illness is curable and does not impede my soul. I shall not lay violent hands upon myself just because I am in pain; for death under such circumstances is defeat. But if I find out that the pain must always be endured, I shall depart, not because of the pain, but because it will be a hindrance to me as regards all my reasons for living.[1]

The advent of Christianity led to great changes in this attitude. For long periods in the history of the Christian Church, seemingly pointless and sometimes grotesque suffering was seen as a burden imposed on us by God Himself, for reasons known only to Him. Life was not our own to be disposed of at will, but a gift from God, which only He had a right to reclaim.

While this has been the prevailing attitude for hundreds of years, it is no longer universally shared. There are many Christian thinkers today – both Catholic and Protestant – who believe that their respective religious frameworks permit an incurably ill person to deliberately end her life. Two of the contributors to this collection, Kenneth Ralph, a Minister of the Uniting Church of Australia, and Max Charlesworth, an Emeritus Professor of Philosophy and a practising Catholic, take this view.

Many of those who subscribe to non-Christian beliefs, or to no religious beliefs at all, agree with the fundamental premise that incurably ill people have a moral right to choose their own death. As has repeatedly been pointed out in this collection, 78 per cent of Australians now believe that doctors should be allowed to end a patient's life, at the patient's request, if the patient is hopelessly ill, in great pain, and has no chance of recovery.[2]

The belief that a hopelessly ill person has a right to die does, however, sit rather uncomfortably with existing laws. For a long time, suicide has been regarded as a most heinous offence against both God and King. As Sir William Blackstone summed it up some 230 years ago in his famous *Commentaries on the Laws of England:* 'The suicide is guilty of a double offence: one spiritual, in invading the prerogative of the Almighty and rushing into His immediate presence uncalled for; the other temporal, against the King, who hath an interest in the preservation of all his subjects.'[3]

In 1961, suicide was decriminalised in England, and the Australian States (with the exception of the Northern Territory) have since followed suit. While attempted suicides are thus no longer subject to punishment under criminal law, assisting someone to end her life remains a criminal offence. A person who helps another to end her life may be charged with the offence of aiding and abetting suicide; a person who ends another's life, at that person's request, may be charged with murder.

The mere fact that an action is unlawful does not, of course, mean that it is morally wrong. On the contrary, sometimes it is the law – not the action – that deserves moral condemnation. Our law, which prohibits direct aid in dying to the incurably ill who request it, is such a law. It enforces behaviour that leads to much unnecessary suffering and unjustifiably restricts the liberty or autonomy of the very people it is meant to protect.

When we are thinking about medically assisted suicide or voluntary euthanasia, two main questions arise. The first question is whether we may sometimes legitimately choose death for ourselves. The second question is whether it is proper for doctors to help us in this quest.

There is widespread agreement amongst those who approach morality from very different ethical or religious perspectives that there are times when it is morally proper for a person to choose death. As autonomous moral agents we may decide to lay down our lives for another person, or for an ideal, and we may even decide that it is best for us, and for those close to us, that we should seek release from a life of illness that has become an intolerable burden to us.

Every contributor to this collection, including Nicholas Tonti-Filippini who approaches questions of death and dying from a traditional Roman Catholic perspective, agrees that life is not an absolute value and that there is no moral obligation to preserve it for as long as possible. Disagreement arises when it comes to the question of how, and by what means, we are morally permitted to bring death about. The traditional view is that patients may legitimately reject burdensome treatment, as Mrs N. in Nick Tonti-Filippini's article did, even if this is known to lead to death. In addition, it is thought that patients who are in great pain may legitimately accept pain-killing drugs and sedation in quantities that are likely to shorten life. What patients are not permitted to do is to directly and intentionally end their lives by, for example, taking a lethal dose of a drug.

Why is this? The view that we must never deliberately cut short our lives might make some sense if one believes that we are the property of God or the King, as Blackstone explained in his *Commentaries on the Laws of England*, or that morality consists in our blindly following a rule that prohibits us from doing so. Most thinkers, including religious thinkers, today reject this view. They believe that morality is not a matter of blind obedience, but rather a matter of reason and autonomous choice.

As Kenneth Ralph has pointed out, it is difficult to conceive of any moral or religious scheme in which the notion of personal autonomy does not occupy a central place. Autonomy – the capacity to think for ourselves, to form, revise and pursue our own plans for life – is basic to our understanding of ethics, and to our self-understanding as persons.

If autonomy is a central moral value, there are good reasons for incorporating it into the public policies of a multicultural and pluralist society like our own. In such a liberal society, Max Charlesworth explains, the right to choose one's own way of life for oneself (and respect for the rights of others to do the same) is the overriding value. This means, of course, that there must be a clear dividing line between the sphere of private morality and the sphere of public policy and the law. People are free to live their own lives, in accordance with their own autonomously chosen values and beliefs, as long as they do not cause harm to others. It would be quite illegitimate to restrict one person's liberty merely because her action conflicts with somebody else's moral code.

This has obvious implications for a person's end-of-life decisions, where harm to others is not an issue. The mere fact that it is wrong, according to some moral views, for an incurably ill person to end her life by direct means is no reason for the law to step in to prevent that person from carrying out her autonomous decision, and to force her to die in a way that is utterly abhorrent to her. Max Charlesworth quotes Ronald Dworkin to amplify this point: 'Making someone die in a way that others approve, but he regards as a horrifying contradiction of his life, is a devastating, odious form of tyranny.'[4]

Yet this frequently happens in our own society. The essays in this collection bear ample witness to this. People are forced to die in ways that they regard as a horrifying contradiction of their lives because the law does not allow them to seek direct help in dying from doctors who are willing to provide it.

It will be said that the charge is misplaced. After all, the law does not prevent anybody from ending her life. Suicide is no longer a crime. Anybody who wants to end her life is free to do so. As a Melbourne psychiatrist once said to me: 'I don't know why there is all this fuss about voluntary euthanasia. People can always commit suicide.' When I pointed out that it was very difficult for anyone, especially the very ill and incapacitated, to do this, she said that if people really wanted to die – which she doubted – they could 'always either jump out of a window or put their fingers into an electric power point.'

Not many incurably ill patients would wish to die in this way and, thankfully, not many health care professionals take so callous an approach. On the contrary, 60 per cent of doctors and 78 per cent of nurses want the law changed so that it will be possible for doctors to lawfully practise voluntary euthanasia – that is, end an incurably ill person's life, at that person's request.[5]

Again, there will be objections. It might be said that it is one thing for a person to commit suicide; helping that person to end her life is quite another. It is difficult to see why this should be so. If it is not wrong for me to end my life under certain circumstances, why should it be wrong for another person, such as a doctor, to help me die?

As has repeatedly been pointed out, helping a suffering person to end her life can be an act of great love. While relatives and friends will frequently perform this last act of love, sometimes at great cost to themselves, many of the articles demonstrate that this is a bad solution. Ending one's life in a painless and dignified way requires not only access to such things as drugs, but also knowledge and skills. As Mary Mortimer writes: 'Fourteen years later, I still feel the rage and despair of being abandoned in our urgent need. That a beloved partner has to die is enough to bear; that enabling him or her to die with dignity should be accompanied by such terror and helplessness is an outrage in a society that considers itself civilised or caring.'

If incurably ill people who want to die are denied lawful assistance to end their lives, they will often be driven to use violent and undignified methods. Unwilling to involve relatives or friends in an unlawful act, they will often die alone. As George Quittner puts it in his commentary on the death of his patient, Chris Hill: 'It was tragic that a man with his disability was denied any assistance with the most important act of his life ... Chris died alone, not by choice, but because he was driven there by an inhumane society. The strident voices who "sanctify life" drove him to an unpleasant death.'

Doctors have the relevant expertise to give advice and to prescribe or administer drugs that would allow patients who cannot be helped in any other way to end their lives in a painless and dignified manner. It would not be contrary to the doctor's role to prescribe or administer such drugs, at the patient's request. Doctors have two primary duties: to respect the autonomy of their patients and to ensure their well-being, through the relief of suffering. As the palliative care specialists Roger Hunt and Pieter Admiraal explain, voluntary euthanasia can be seen as an appropriate part of proper patient care; under some circumstances, it is the last and most dignified act that a doctor can perform for a patient when all else has failed. There are even occasions, the Melbourne specialist Rodney Syme suggests, when it would be an 'unforgivable act of cowardice and inhumanity – an immoral act,' to deny a patient direct help in dying.

Our laws relating to medical treatment implicitly recognise that it would not only be inhumane, but also contrary to the principle of autonomy or bodily self-determination, to impose on patients a life they do not want. Competent patients are able to refuse life-sustaining treatment, and to request adequate palliative care, even if this will shorten life. This has implications for the role of doctors. Doctors are legally permitted, even required, to turn off life-sustaining machines and to discontinue other treatments that keep patients alive, if this is what the informed patient wants. It is probably also lawful, although there is still some dispute about this, for doctors to administer pain relief and sedation in quantities that are likely to shorten life. All this is considered part of good medical practice, of good patient care. But if it is lawful for patients and doctors to shorten life in these 'indirect' ways, why should it be unlawful for patients and doctors to make another kind of life-shortening decision – one that will directly end life and give patients the kind of dignified death they want?

There are a number of reasons, all of them explicitly or implicitly contained in this collection, why doctors should be allowed to assist the dying in more direct ways than the law currently permits them to do. They concern respect for autonomy, the duty to minimise suffering, and the issue of unjust discrimination.

When a patient refuses treatment, death will not always come quickly and painlessly. Refusal of treatment can result in a drawn-out and very unpleasant death. Every health care professional knows this, and every honest health care professional will admit it.

Now, if a fully informed patient wishes to die by refusal of treatment, as Mrs N. appears to have done, this is a decision that we should respect, and generally much can be done to ease the patient's passing. This does not, however, answer the question of why we should not equally respect the choices of a person who is horrified and appalled by the idea that she must die slowly and in what she regards as an undignified manner of 'natural causes', and would like to end her life in a direct way. For the purposes of public policy the two decisions ought to be the same: in dialogue with the doctor, the fully informed patient decides on a course of action that will lead to a dignified death, and the doctor assists her in carrying it out. The mere fact that some people regard instances of the direct termination of life as morally wrong is no reason, in a liberal society, to deny those who do not share this view access to other ways of ending their lives.

One might even claim that our laws are discriminatory. John McEwan, one of the patients described in Nick Tonti-Filippini's article, wished to die. So did Cornelis Hus, whose case Janine Hosking describes. Both had sustained severe injuries and were now quadriplegic. A person in John McEwan's position is able to lawfully implement his wish to die, whereas a person in Cornelis Hus's position is condemned to a life that he does not want. Why? Not because one person has formed a stronger and more autonomous desire to die, nor because one person suffers more than the other, but because of a consideration that ought to be utterly irrelevant: that one person does, and the other person does not, require life-support.

A law which says that a patient who suffers from quadriplegia and happens to require life-support is permitted to end his life, with the help of doctors, whereas another person who is also quadriplegic but does not happen to require life-support, is not permitted to do so, is discriminatory. It discriminates against those who want to die, but who are not 'fortunate' enough to require life-support.[6]

There is another interesting way in which the charge of discrimination might be raised. If it is not unlawful for an able-bodied person to end her life, it might be argued that a law which prevents a severely disabled person from obtaining help from others to do the same is discriminatory. Such a case was recently taken to the Supreme Court of Canada by Sue Rodriguez, a woman who (like Mrs N. in Nick Tonti-Filippini's example) was suffering from motor neurone disease. Her argument was this: as long as she was still able to do certain things for herself, her life was valuable to her and she did not want to die. But, because the disease was incurable and progressive, she would soon be totally disabled. It would be then that she would wish to die. By that stage, though, she would no longer be able to take her own life. Because Canadian law prohibits assisted suicide, Sue Rodriguez argued that it unjustly prevented a disabled person like herself from getting help in doing what an able-bodied person can lawfully do without help. The Supreme Court ruled against her – but only by a slim 5 to 4 majority vote – and the outcome might easily have been different.[7]

Finally, we come to the topic of palliative care. As has repeatedly been noted by contributors to this collection, modern palliative care is a very positive development. It allows many people to die with dignity. Very often pain can be controlled or relieved, and symptom control has been much improved. But the best of palliative care cannot, as the palliative care specialists Roger Hunt and Pieter Admiraal have pointed out, help all patients. The reason is not, or not only, that there are some instances when pain cannot be controlled (other than through rendering the patient permanently unconscious), but rather and more fundamentally that pain is not the central issue. The central issue is one of dignity. A dignified death is a death that accords with the patient's values and beliefs, a death that does not contradict the patient's life. A death that is imposed by the moral or religious beliefs of others is not a dignified death – even if it is relatively pain-free. As Max Charlesworth has noted, if one takes the values and beliefs of others seriously, then one will focus not so much on a pain-free or 'happy death', but on an autonomous death. Mary Mortimer puts this into context when she writes of her husband, Rex: 'He greatly feared losing his dignity, indeed "losing his mind". He was afraid that the end of his life would be humiliating, and that our memory of him would be of a sick, incapable, irrational "patient", rather than the full human being he was in our lives.'

Because the central issue is one of dignity, of respect for the patient's values and beliefs, palliative care can never meet the needs of all patients. Chris Hill's powerful contribution to this book makes this point more clearly and convincingly than any number of philosophical arguments ever could.

There are various reasons why our existing laws seem untenable: because they unjustifiably deny people's liberty, forcing them to die in ways which cause unnecessary suffering and which they regard as undignified and as a contradiction of their lives, and because these laws discriminate against the disabled, and against those who do not require life-support.

Not many people today would want to claim that we must uphold the prohibition of medically assisted suicide (where the doctor prescribes the drugs that the patient may take to end her life) and volunary euthanasia (where the doctor ends the patient's life, at the patient's request) simply because helping the patient die in this way is contrary to some private moral or religious code. Rather, opponents of assisted dying and voluntary euthanasia, even if motivated by such views, will typically rely on a different and more universal claim.They grant that direct help in dying may benefit some patients, but claim that allowing doctors to provide it will lead to greater harm to others. The type of reasoning appealed to here is the 'slippery slope argument', which asserts that some morally good or morally neutral practices will have such bad consequences that they must not be allowed. With regard to medically assisted suicide or voluntary euthanasia, it is usually claimed that once doctors are allowed to end the lives of the incurably ill who want to die, it won't be long before they will engage in the killing of other patients – those who are neither terminally ill, nor want to die.

If correct, this argument stemming from harm to others would be a strong reason for retaining laws that will prevent doctors from providing direct aid in dying. Harm to others is, as Max Charlesworth has pointed out and as I have reiterated, the only consideration that can legitimately be invoked in a liberal society to override the autonomy and freedom of some of its members.

Is this argument sound? And what evidence could be produced to back up the claim that doctors who take the autonomy and the suffering of their patients so seriously that they are not only prepared to 'allow' them to die, but are actually prepared to help them die, will turn into indiscriminate killers? A closer look at the arguments will show that there is no evidence at all.

People who oppose the decriminalisation or legalisation of medically assisted suicide and voluntary euthanasia will often refer to the so-called 'euthanasia' program of the Nazis and cite it as an example of what can happen when a society acknowledges that there are some lives which are so compromised that they may deliberately be taken. But this example cannot back up the argument. The motivation behind Hitler's 'euthanasia' program was neither respect for the autonomy of the people who were killed, nor empathy for their suffering; it was rather racial prejudice and the belief that the purity of the *Volk* required the elimination of certain individuals and groups.

More recently, opponents of medically assisted dying have pointed to the Netherlands in support of the claim that doctors must not be allowed to provide direct help in dying to their patients. Although assisted suicide is not everywhere a crime (it is, for example, lawful in Switzerland, Germany, and the American state of Michigan), the Netherlands is currently the only country in the world which allows doctors to also practise voluntary euthanasia.

A Dutch study on euthanasia and other medical end-of-life decisions known as the Remmelink Report[8], which was published in 1991, is thought to confirm that the decriminalisation of voluntary euthanasia in the Netherlands has had some very undesirable consquences. But this conclusion is either based on some very muddled thinking or on a deliberate distortion of facts.[9]

The Remmelink Report, probably the largest and most sophisticated study of medical end-of-life decisions published anywhere in the world, is interesting for a number of reasons. It shows, for example, that the practice of euthanasia and medically assisted suicide is relatively rare. Active euthanasia occurred in 2.6 per cent of all deaths, and assisted suicide in 0.3 per cent. Thirty-five per cent of deaths, however, were the result of two other kinds of medical end-of-life decision: 17.5 per cent of patients died because treatment was withheld or withdrawn, and 17.5 per cent died because they were given potentially life-shortening palliative care. Now, if one is worried about slippery slopes and abuse, would it not be much more reasonable - in terms of the absolute numbers involved and hence the possible scope for abuse - to worry about the last two types of end-of-life decisions, rather than about the relatively small number of cases where death resulted from a direct intervention? It seems the answer ought to be yes.

This morally or religiously motivated focus on some end-of-life decisions, to the neglect of others, is not the central question when one wants to use a large-scale study, such as the Remmelink Report, to prove or disprove the existence of a slippery slope. Rather the question is this: Can an extensive empirical study, whatever its findings, confirm or deny the existence of a slippery slope?

In 1992, one doctor wrote in the *Medical Journal of Australia* that '[t]he disturbing statistics from the Remmelink Report indicate that doctors and the community should emphatically reject any moves to legalize similar practices in Australia'[10]; and a researcher in the field of bioethics wrote that the evidence from the Netherlands 'now available in the official Dutch reports ... provides conclusive evidence of the slippery slope ... '[11] But these conclusions do not follow. The reason for this is rather simple.

To demonstrate the existence of a slippery slope, one would

need to show that a society is worse off after introducing a new practice. In other words, one would have to prove that there are now more unjustified deaths in the Netherlands than there were before doctors could openly provide direct aid in dying. Since the Remmelink Report is the first large-scale study of its kind, no such figures are available. This means that no legitimate conclusions about the existence (or non-existence) of a slippery slope can be drawn from the figures found in the report. There may have been more, or fewer, cases of unjustifiable termination of life in the Netherlands before the decriminalisation of voluntary euthanasia. We simply don't know.

Nor do we know how the numbers of various medical end-of-life decisions in the Netherlands compare with medical end-of-life decisions in other countries, including our own. What we do know, however, is that medical end-of-life decisions are also made in Australia. For example, even though doctors are not permitted to practise voluntary euthanasia in Australia, two studies suggest that more than 25 per cent of doctors who have been asked to do so by a patient have, in fact, directly ended a patient's life.[12] But we do not know how many patients in Australia die because treatment is withdrawn, or because their lives are shortened by the administration of palliative care, nor do we know – surely the central concern – how many of those able to do so did not give their consent. This means that no qualitative and quantitive comparisons between the Netherlands and countries such as our own are possible. Contrary to what some opponents of voluntary euthanasia think, there could well be a greater incidence of unconsented-to medical end-of-life decisions in countries like ours, where open decision-making and dialogue between doctors and patients is not permitted, than in the Netherlands, which freely acknowledges that direct aid in dying must sometimes be part of good medical practice.

How does the Netherlands regulate the practice of medically assisted suicide and voluntary euthanasia? According to the Dutch Penal Code, voluntary euthanasia and assisted suicide, even if practised by doctors, is unlawful. Since 1973, Dutch courts have, however, developed case law according to which doctors (and only doctors) will not be prosecuted if they observe the following five principles:

1 there must be a free and voluntary request from the patient;
2 the request must be well-informed and well-considered;
3 the request must be durable;
4 the patient must experience unacceptable suffering which cannot satisfactorily be relieved;
5 the doctor must consult with a (senior) colleague.

In their reasoning, the courts have appealed to the legal doctrine of 'force majeure', that is, to a principle of necessity which compels a person to choose between two incompatible duties or obligations. A doctor who is caring for an incurably ill and suffering patient who wants to die is, in this view, faced by two conflicting duties: the professional duty to respect the patient's wish to die, and the civil duty to respect the laws of the land. Since doctors cannot fulfil both duties, the reasoning is that doctors, who put their professional duty to their patients first, cannot be held responsible for failing to fulfil their duty as citizens.

A doctor who has performed voluntary euthanasia or assisted suicide is then required to provide comprehensive details of the circumstances of the case to the local medical examiner who, in turn, will report to the public prosecutor. The public prosecutor will then decide whether all the conditions have been satisfied or whether the doctor should be prosecuted.

This notification procedure for cases of voluntary euthanasia and assisted suicide has recently been incorporated into an amendment to the Dutch Burial Act and has thus been given statutory authority.

There is some debate about the notification procedure itself, which is sometimes seen as excessively bureaucratic and cumbersome and therefore thought to be discouraging doctors from reporting all cases of voluntary euthanasia and assisted suicide. This may or may not be the case. Procedural matters, while not unimportant, do not go to the heart of the matter. The basic question is whether those who are terminally or incurably ill should be able to lawfully enlist the help of willing doctors to end their lives – either by prescribing a dose of a drug, or by providing direct help in dying. Once that question has been answered in the affirmative, it will not be beyond the capabilities of modern societies to devise procedures and frameworks that will protect the rights of patients who want to die, the interests of doctors who are willing to listen, and the rights and interests of all those who want to live their lives in accordance with some other values or beliefs.

In Victoria, for example, it might be a relatively simple matter to extend the *Medical Treatment Act 1988*, to allow not only refusal of treatment by competent patients, but also direct help in dying. Safeguards are already in place to protect patients from abuse, and doctors against unwarranted legal interference. The same safeguards could cover cases where life is terminated not by 'indirect', but by direct means.

Another way in which our society might decide to proceed is to uphold the current prohibition on voluntary euthanasia, while decriminalising medically assisted suicide. This is proposed in legislation – the Medical Treatment (Assistance to the Dying) Bill 1993 – promulgated by the Voluntary Euthanasia Society of Victoria. This Bill would allow doctors to provide terminally ill patients with the means to end their lives. While the Bill might not help every patient, and would fall short of the freely available 'little black pill' envisaged by

Terry Lane, it would be a first step towards liberalising laws that unjustifiably prevent doctors and patients from jointly deciding on one of a range of possible end-of-life options that best meets the needs of the patient.

The absence of a legal framework does not mean that doctors will refrain from practising voluntary euthanasia, or refrain from helping some of their desperately ill patients commit suicide. It merely means that many doctors will, at potentially great cost to themselves, be breaking the law, to assist their patients to die in ways that they regard as morally and professionally sound.

As we have noted, two recent surveys indicate that more than a quarter of doctors engaged in the care of incurably or terminally ill adult patients have practised voluntary euthanasia at least once.[12] A doctor who directly ends a patient's life, at the patient's request, may be charged with murder; and a doctor who prescribes or provides drugs for the patient to take may be charged with the crime of 'aiding and abetting' a suicide.

These doctors should not be subject to criminal sanctions in a liberal society such as ours. They are not committing crimes, rather they are acting in accordance with the widely accepted professional and moral principles that doctors have a duty to respect their patients' autonomy and a duty to alleviate their suffering. Of course, they are doing so in 'direct' ways, rather than in the 'indirect' ways (withdrawal of treatment and life-shortening palliative care) sanctioned by our society. But the distinction between 'direct' and 'indirect' ways of aiding a patient's dying deserves no place in the legal framework of a liberal society.

Besides, even though there is little doubt that doctors are ordinarily acting from the highest of motives when they are providing direct aid in dying to their patients, it is rather unsatisfactory that they should be making these end-of-life decisions without any public guidance, and without any public scrutiny. To knowingly leave it to doctors to perform 'criminal actions' means that we are imposing on them a burden which they should not have to bear on their own.

For a number of reasons, the honest and open Dutch approach is very much preferable to our own. Patients can lawfully request direct help in dying from doctors willing to provide it; Dutch doctors do not have to fear legal sanctions if they abide by the patient's request, and Dutch society as a whole has accepted responsibility for the implementation of procedural frameworks that will protect patients and doctors alike. We have yet to accept that responsibility.

One thing is certain, though. Without a change in our legal framework Australian doctors will not be able to truly listen to those who want to die – and patients will be dying in ways that are a horrible contradiction of their lives. Those who have told their sometimes painful stories in this collection have spoken for many others. I thank them, on behalf of all of us.

NOTES

1. Seneca, '58th Letter to Lucilius', trans. R. M. Gummere, in T. E. Page et al. (eds) *Seneca: Ad Lucilium Epistulae Morales*, vol. i, Heinemann, London, 1961, p. 409.

2. Morgan Poll, May 1993, Finding No. 2436.

3. Sir William Blackstone, *Commentaries on the Laws of England*, IV, p. 189, as quoted by Mary Rose Barrington, 'The Case for Rational Suicide' in *Voluntary Euthanasia – Experts Debate the Right to Die*, A. B. Downing and Barbara Smoker (eds), Peter Owen, London, 1986, p. 231.

4. Ronald Dworkin, *Life's Dominion; An Argument about Abortion, Euthanasia and Individual Freedom*, Knopf, New York, 1993.

5. Helga Kuhse and Peter Singer, 'Doctors' practices and attitudes regarding voluntary euthanasia', *Medical Journal of Australia*, vol. 148, 20 June 1988, pp. 623–27; Helga Kuhse and Peter Singer: 'Voluntary euthanasia and the nurse: An Australian Survey', *International Journal of Nursing Studies*, vol. 30, no. 4, 1993, pp. 311–22.

6. It is an interesting ethical and legal question whether a person who refuses treatment because she wants to die is committing suicide. If this were the case, it would be unlawful for a doctor to discontinue treatment – because the doctor would then be assisting in a suicide.

7. *Sue Rodriguez v. The Attorney General of Canada and the Attorney General of British Columbia*, Supreme Court of Canada, File No. 23476; 30 September, 1993. See also *Monash Bioethics Review*, vol. 13, no. 1, January 1994, pp. 11–12.

8. P. J. van der Maas, J. J. M. van Delden, L. Pijnenborg, *Medische Beslissen Rond het, Levenseinde*, Erasmus University, Rotterdam, 1991; P. J. van der Maas, J. J. M. van Delden, L. Pijnenborg, C. W. N. Looman, 'Euthanasia and other medical decisions concerning the end of life', *The Lancet*, vol. 338, 14 Sept. 1991, pp. 669–74. (While these findings are typically referred to as the 'Remmelink Report', this is, strictly, not correct. The Remmelink Report was produced on the basis of those investigations and contained recommendations to the Dutch government. Because the investigation of P. J. van der Maas and his colleagues are, however, so widely known in Australia as the 'Remmelink Report', I have continued to use the term.)

9. See Helga Kuhse, 'Voluntary Euthanasia in the Netherlands and Slippery Slopes, *Bioethics News*, vol. 11, no. 4, July 1992, pp. 1–7.

10. G. D. Tracy, 'Medical aspects of Euthanasia', *Medical Journal of Australia*, vol. 156, 1992, pp. 579–80.

11. J. I. Fleming, 'Euthanasia, the Netherlands and slippery slopes', *Bioethics Research Notes*, Supplement 4 (2), 1992.

12. H. Kuhse and P. Singer, 'Doctors' practices and attitudes regarding voluntary euthanasia', op. cit. (This study has been repeated by the Department of Community Medicine of the University of New South Wales. At the time of writing, only one figure had been released: that 'more than a quarter' of doctors surveyed who were treating terminally ill or incurably ill patients and had been asked to do so had deliberately ended the patient's life. In the Kuhse/Singer survey, the figure was 29 per cent.)

13. ibid.

Recommended
Further Reading

Barnard, Christiaan, *Good Life – Good Death. A Doctor's Case for Euthanasia and Suicide*, Prentice Hall, Englewood Cliffs, NJ, 1980.

Brook, Dan W., *Life and Death – Philosophical Essays in Biomedical Ethics*, Cambridge University Press, Cambridge, 1993.

Campbell, Robert and Collinson, Diane, *Ending Lives*, Basic Blackwell, Oxford, 1988.

Donnelly, John (ed.), *Suicide – Right or Wrong?* Prometheus Books, Buffalo, NY, 1990.

Downing, A. B. and Smoker, Barbara (eds), *Voluntary Euthanasia – Experts Debate the Right to Die*, Peter Owen, London, 1986.

Fletcher, Joseph, *Humanhood: Essays in Biomedical Ethics*, Prometheus Books, Buffalo, NY, 1979.

Harris, John, *The Value of Life – An Introduction to Medical Ethics*, Routledge & Kegan Paul, London, 1985.

Humphry, Derek, *Final Exit – The practicalities of self-deliverance and assisted suicide for the dying* (Australian edition prepared by Helga Kuhse), Penguin Books, Ringwood, Vic., 1991.

Humphry, Derek and Wickett, Ann, *The Right to Die – Understanding Euthanasia*, Harper & Row, New York, 1986.

Humphry, Derek and Wickett, Ann, *Jean's Way*, The Hemlock Society, Eugene, Oregon, reprinted 1991.

Kennedy, Ludovic, *Euthanasia – The Good Death*, Chatto & Windus, London, 1990.

Kuhse, Helga, *The Sanctity-of-Life Doctrine in Medicine – A Critique*, Oxford University Press, Oxford, 1987.

Kuhse, Helga and Singer, Peter, *Individuals, Humans, Persons: Questions of Life and Death*, Academia Verlag, Sankt Angustin, 1994.

Lanham, David, *Taming Death by Law*, Longman Professional Publishing, Melbourne, 1993.

Mackay, John (ed.), *Active Voluntary Euthanasia – The Current Issues, Proceedings of a Conference organized by the Centre for Human Bioethics, Monash University – Royal Australasian College of Surgeons, November 15, 1993*, Monash University Centre for Human Bioethics, Melbourne, 1994.

Rachels, James, *The End of Life – Euthanasia and Morality*, Oxford University Press, Oxford, 1986.

Rollin, Betty, *Last Wish*, Signet, New York, 1987.

Social Development Committee, Parliament of Victoria, *First Report on Inquiry into Options for Dying with Dignity – Incorporating a Discussion Paper: A Range of Views on Options for Dying with Dignity*, Government Printer, Melbourne, 1986.

Social Development Committee, Parliament of Victoria, *Inquiry into Options for Dying with Dignity – Second and Final Report*, Government Printer, Melbourne, 1987.

Wennberg, Robert N., *Terminal Choices – Euthanasia, Suicide and the Right to Die*, William B. Eerdmans Publishing Company, Grand Rapids, Michigan, and The Paternoster Press, Exeter, UK, 1989.

Australian and New Zealand Voluntary Euthanasia Societies

Many countries now have active 'right to die' movements. In Australia, there are currently ten voluntary euthanasia societies, and New Zealand has two. The reason for the high number of Australian societies is that all are trying to achieve law reform, and law reform is a State matter.

Strength comes from numbers. If you, the reader of this book, think that the time for legislative change has come, you might wish to join your State voluntary euthanasia society, thereby helping this change to come about.

AUSTRALIAN SOCIETIES
Victoria
Voluntary Euthanasia Society of Victoria Inc. (VESV)
70 Greville St
Prahran, Vic. 3181
Tel. (03) 521 3297
Fax (03) 521 3302

New South Wales
Voluntary Euthanasia Society of NSW Inc.
PO Box 25
Broadway, NSW 2007
Tel. (02) 212 4782

South Australia
South Australian Voluntary Euthanasia Society Inc. (SAVES)
PO Box 2151
Kent Town Centre, SA 5071
Tel. (08) 379 3421

Western Australia
West Australian Voluntary Euthanasia Society Inc. (WAVES)
PO Box 7243
Cloisters Square
Perth, WA 6001
Tel. (09) 367 6483

Queensland
Brisbane
Voluntary Euthanasia Society of Queensland (VESQ)
PO Box 10204
Brisbane, Qld 4001
Tel. (07) 882 1139

Cairns
Voluntary Euthanasia Society of Queensland (Cairns Branch)
PO Box 175
Cairns, Qld 4870
Tel. (070) 53 1486

Tasmania
Voluntary Euthanasia Society of Tasmania
PO Box 8
Irishtown, Tas. 7330
Tel. (004) 56 1344

Voluntary Euthanasia Society of Tasmania
(Northern Branch)
C/- Mr T. Hague
Hillwood, Tas. 7252
Tel. (003) 94 8131

Voluntary Euthanasia Society of Southern Tasmania (VEST)
PO Box 47
North Hobart, Tas. 7002
Tel. (002) 732 853

ACT
Voluntary Euthanasia Society of New South Wales Inc.
(Canberra Branch)
PO Box 4029
Kingston, ACT 2604
Tel. (06) 295 9412

NEW ZEALAND SOCIETIES
Auckland
Voluntary Euthanasia Society (Auckland) Inc.
PO Box 3709
Auckland

Wellington
Voluntary Euthanasia Society
95 Melrose Rd
Island Bay, Wellington
Tel. 383 7752

Index

INDEX